Congestive Heart Failure Diet Cookbook

A Comprehensive Cookbook for Managing Congestive Heart Failure with Flavorful Wellness and Sustaining Heart Health

Silvia Carroll

Table of Content

A strong heart is the foundation of a strong life.

Introduction

I'm Dr. Silvia Carroll, and I'm thrilled to welcome you to the "Congestive Heart Failure Diet Cookbook." With over 15 years of experience in the field of cardiovascular health, it's my privilege to share this collection of recipes and insights with you.

Throughout my career, I've dedicated myself to understanding the intricate relationship between diet and heart health. Witnessing the impact of nutrition on individuals managing congestive heart failure has fueled my commitment to creating a resource that goes beyond mere recipes. This cookbook is a culmination of my knowledge, passion, and the belief that a heart-healthy lifestyle can be both achievable and enjoyable.

In these pages, you'll find more than just a list of ingredients and cooking instructions. Each recipe is a reflection of my dedication to providing nourishing, flavorful options that align with the unique dietary considerations of those with congestive heart failure.

Whether you're taking your first steps toward managing your heart health or looking to enhance your existing practices, consider this cookbook your companion on the journey. I invite you to explore, savor, and embrace the joy of delicious, heart-conscious meals.

Here's to your health and the fulfilling journey toward a heart-healthy

Understanding Congestive Heart Failure

Congestive Heart Failure (CHF) is an intricate cardiovascular condition characterized by the heart's inability to pump blood effectively, leading to compromised circulation and insufficient oxygen delivery to the body's tissues. This condition, while chronic, can be managed with a comprehensive understanding of its mechanisms, symptoms, diagnostic processes, and treatment approaches.

Symptoms of Congestive Heart Failure:

Symptoms of Congestive Heart Failure (CHF) can vary, and individuals may experience a combination of the following signs, indicating a compromised ability of the heart to pump blood effectively:

Shortness of Breath (Dyspnea): Difficulty breathing, especially during physical activities or when lying down, is a common symptom. This can be due to fluid accumulation in the lungs.

Persistent Coughing: Individuals with CHF may have a chronic cough that produces white or pink-tinged phlegm. This occurs when fluid backs up into the lungs.

Fatigue and Weakness: Reduced blood flow to vital organs can result in persistent fatigue and a general feeling of weakness, impacting daily activities.

Fluid Retention (Edema): Swelling in the legs, ankles, and abdomen is a noticeable symptom. It occurs when the heart's pumping efficiency decreases, causing fluid to accumulate in the body.

Rapid or Irregular Heartbeat: Heart palpitations or an irregular pulse may be experienced. This can be a result of the heart's struggle to maintain a normal rhythm.

Increased Heart Rate (Tachycardia): The heart may beat faster than normal, especially during physical exertion or as a compensatory mechanism for reduced cardiac output.

Reduced Exercise Tolerance: Individuals with CHF may find it challenging to engage in physical activities they could previously handle without difficulty.

Difficulty Sleeping: The accumulation of fluid in the lungs can lead to nighttime coughing and breathlessness, causing disruptions in sleep patterns.

Sudden Weight Gain: Unexplained weight gain, often accompanied by swelling, can be indicative of fluid retention associated with CHF.

Loss of Appetite or Nausea: CHF can affect the digestive system, leading to a diminished appetite, feelings of fullness, or nausea.

These symptoms may vary in severity, and not everyone with CHF will experience all of them. Additionally, symptoms may develop gradually or suddenly, depending on the underlying cause and progression of the condition.

Types of Congestive Heart Failure:

Congestive Heart Failure (CHF) can manifest in different types based on which side of the heart is primarily affected and the specific dysfunction present. The main types of CHF are as follows:

- Left-Sided Heart Failure:

Systolic Heart Failure: In this type, the left ventricle of the heart is weakened and cannot pump blood effectively, leading to reduced circulation of oxygenated blood to the body.

Diastolic Heart Failure: The left ventricle becomes stiff and cannot relax properly during the heart's resting phase (diastole), hindering the heart's ability to fill with blood.

- Right-Sided Heart Failure:

This occurs when the right ventricle is unable to pump blood efficiently to the lungs for oxygenation. It often follows left-sided heart failure but can also result from lung-related conditions.

- Combined or Biventricular Heart Failure:

In some cases, both the left and right sides of the heart are affected simultaneously, leading to combined or biventricular heart failure. This results in a comprehensive impairment of the heart's pumping function.

- High-Output Heart Failure:

This less common type of CHF is characterized by hyperdynamic circulation where the heart pumps a larger-than-normal volume of blood but still fails to meet the body's demands. It can be caused by conditions such as anemia, hyperthyroidism, or arteriovenous fistulas.

- Low-Output Heart Failure:

In contrast to high-output heart failure, low-output heart failure occurs when the heart's pumping capacity is diminished, leading to insufficient blood circulation. This is a more typical presentation of CHF.

Causes of Congestive Heart Failure:
Congestive Heart Failure (CHF) can arise from various underlying conditions that affect the heart's ability to pump blood effectively. Understanding the causes is crucial for identifying risk factors and implementing preventive measures. Here are common causes of Congestive Heart Failure:

- Coronary Artery Disease (CAD):

The most prevalent cause of CHF, CAD occurs when the coronary arteries that supply blood to the heart muscle become narrowed or blocked, restricting blood flow and leading to heart muscle damage.

- Myocardial Infarction (Heart Attack):

A heart attack can result in permanent damage to the heart muscle, impairing its ability to contract and pump blood adequately.

- Hypertension (High Blood Pressure):

Prolonged high blood pressure forces the heart to work harder to pump blood against increased resistance. Over time, this can lead to heart muscle thickening and weakening.

- Cardiomyopathy:

Conditions that directly affect the heart muscle, such as dilated cardiomyopathy, hypertrophic cardiomyopathy, or restrictive cardiomyopathy, can contribute to CHF.

- Valvular Heart Diseases:

Malfunctioning heart valves, such as aortic stenosis or mitral regurgitation, can disrupt blood flow, leading to heart failure.

- Myocarditis:

Inflammation of the heart muscle, often caused by viral infections or autoimmune diseases, can weaken the heart and contribute to CHF.

- Congenital Heart Defects:

Structural abnormalities present at birth can lead to heart failure over time.

- Arrhythmias (Irregular Heartbeat):

Persistent irregularities in heart rhythm, especially if rapid or chaotic, can compromise the heart's pumping efficiency.

- Diabetes:

Uncontrolled diabetes can damage blood vessels and contribute to the development of heart disease, increasing the risk of CHF.

- Obesity:

Excess body weight puts additional strain on the heart, increasing the likelihood of heart failure.

- Chronic Lung Diseases:

Conditions such as chronic obstructive pulmonary disease (COPD) can strain the heart, leading to CHF.

- Alcohol and Substance Abuse:

Excessive alcohol consumption and certain illicit substances can contribute to heart muscle damage and heart failure.

- Sleep Apnea:

Untreated sleep apnea, characterized by interruptions in breathing during sleep, is associated with an increased risk of heart failure.

Diagnostic Procedures:

Diagnosing Congestive Heart Failure (CHF) involves a series of diagnostic procedures aimed at assessing the heart's structure, function, and overall health. Healthcare professionals use a combination of tests to confirm the diagnosis and determine the underlying cause. Here are common diagnostic procedures for CHF:

- Echocardiogram:

This non-invasive imaging test uses sound waves to create detailed images of the heart's chambers, valves, and overall function. It helps evaluate the pumping efficiency and identify structural abnormalities.

- Electrocardiogram (ECG or EKG):

An ECG records the electrical activity of the heart, providing information about heart rhythm and detecting irregularities, such as arrhythmias or signs of a previous heart attack.

- Chest X-ray:

X-rays of the chest can reveal the size and shape of the heart. Enlargement of the heart chambers or fluid buildup in the lungs (pulmonary congestion) may be visible.

- Blood Tests:

Blood tests measure specific substances that can indicate heart failure, such as B-type natriuretic peptide (BNP) or N-terminal pro-B-type natriuretic peptide (NT-proBNP). Elevated levels of these markers suggest heart stress or damage.

- Cardiac MRI (Magnetic Resonance Imaging):

This imaging technique provides detailed images of the heart's structure and function. It is particularly useful for assessing the extent of damage to the heart muscle.

- Cardiac CT (Computed Tomography):

CT scans of the heart can help visualize coronary arteries, heart valves, and overall cardiac anatomy. It may be used to identify blockages or abnormalities.

- Stress Test:

Stress tests assess how the heart performs under physical stress. Exercise stress tests involve walking on a treadmill or using medication to stimulate the heart while monitoring heart rate, blood pressure, and ECG changes.

- Holter Monitor or Event Monitor:

These portable devices record continuous or intermittent ECG over 24 hours or longer. They help capture irregular heart rhythms that may not be evident during a standard ECG.

- Nuclear Stress Test:

A nuclear stress test involves injecting a small amount of radioactive material into the bloodstream to assess blood flow to the heart muscle during rest and stress. It provides information about areas with reduced blood supply.

- Coronary Angiography:

This invasive procedure involves injecting contrast dye into the coronary arteries and taking X-ray images. It helps identify blockages or narrowing in the arteries that supply blood to the heart.

- Biopsy:

In some cases, a small tissue sample (biopsy) from the heart muscle may be taken to assess for inflammatory or infiltrative conditions.

These diagnostic procedures are essential for healthcare professionals to accurately diagnose Congestive Heart Failure, determine its severity, and develop a comprehensive treatment plan tailored to the individual's specific condition. The choice of tests depends on the patient's symptoms, medical history, and clinical presentation.

Importance of a Heart-Healthy Diet

Maintaining a heart-healthy diet is paramount in promoting overall cardiovascular well-being and plays a pivotal role in preventing and managing Congestive Heart Failure (CHF). The importance of adopting dietary practices conducive to heart health cannot be overstated, as these choices directly impact the risk factors associated with heart disease. Here are key reasons highlighting the significance of a heart-healthy diet:

Reducing Risk Factors:

A heart-healthy diet helps manage and control risk factors for heart disease, such as high blood pressure, high cholesterol levels, and obesity. By addressing these factors, individuals can significantly lower their risk of developing CHF.

Managing Blood Pressure:

Sodium intake directly influences blood pressure. A heart-healthy diet emphasizes low-sodium choices, which aid in maintaining optimal blood pressure levels, reducing strain on the heart, and minimizing the risk of heart failure.

Controlling Cholesterol Levels:

A diet rich in fruits, vegetables, whole grains, and healthy fats helps control cholesterol levels. This is crucial in preventing the buildup of plaque in the arteries, reducing the risk of coronary artery disease, and subsequently, heart failure.

Maintaining a Healthy Weight:

Adopting a balanced and nutritious diet contributes to weight management. Maintaining a healthy weight reduces the workload on the heart, preventing excessive strain and lowering the risk of heart failure.

Balancing Blood Sugar Levels:

For individuals with diabetes, a heart-healthy diet is essential in managing blood sugar levels. Diabetes is a significant risk factor for heart disease, and proper dietary choices contribute to overall glycemic control.

Supporting Cardiovascular Function:

Nutrient-rich foods provide essential vitamins and minerals that support optimal cardiovascular function. These nutrients contribute to the health of blood vessels, heart muscles, and overall cardiac performance.

Reducing Inflammation:

Chronic inflammation is associated with various heart conditions. A diet rich in anti-inflammatory foods, such as fruits, vegetables, and omega-3 fatty acids, helps mitigate inflammation, promoting a healthier cardiovascular system.

Optimizing Fluid Balance:

Congestive Heart Failure often involves fluid retention. A heart-healthy diet with controlled sodium intake helps regulate fluid balance, reducing the likelihood of edema and congestion.

Promoting Overall Well-Being:

A heart-healthy diet is not only beneficial for the heart but also for the entire body. It supports overall well-being, providing energy, sustaining vital organs, and enhancing the body's ability to function optimally.

Enhancing Quality of Life:

Adopting a heart-healthy diet contributes to an improved quality of life. It empowers individuals to actively participate in their health, manage chronic conditions effectively, and enjoy a more active and fulfilling lifestyle.

In summary, the importance of a heart-healthy diet extends beyond preventing heart disease; it is a fundamental aspect of maintaining cardiovascular health and preventing the onset or progression of conditions like Congestive Heart Failure. By making informed dietary choices, individuals can take significant steps toward preserving their heart health and overall well-being.

Chapter 1: Nutritional Essentials

In the journey towards heart health and the management of Congestive Heart Failure (CHF), understanding and implementing nutritional essentials is a foundational step. This chapter delves into the crucial role that proper nutrition plays in promoting cardiovascular well-being, providing valuable insights into the key components of a heart-healthy diet.

1.1 Key Nutrients for Heart Health

Achieving and maintaining heart health involves a focus on key nutrients that play crucial roles in supporting cardiovascular function. Understanding the significance of these nutrients empowers individuals in adopting a heart-healthy lifestyle. This section explores essential nutrients and their impact on heart health.

Omega-3 Fatty Acids

Sources:
- Fatty Fish (salmon, mackerel, sardines)
- Flaxseeds and Chia Seeds
- Walnuts
- Algal Oil (for plant-based options)

Role in Heart Health:

Omega-3 fatty acids, particularly EPA and DHA, contribute to cardiovascular health by reducing inflammation, improving lipid profiles, and supporting overall heart function. These essential fats are associated with a lower risk of coronary heart disease.

Antioxidants and Vitamins

Sources:

- Berries (blueberries, strawberries, raspberries)
- Dark Leafy Greens (spinach, kale)
- Nuts and Seeds
- Citrus Fruits (oranges, grapefruits)
- Vegetables (bell peppers, tomatoes)

Role in Heart Health:

Antioxidants, including vitamins C and E, play a vital role in protecting the heart from oxidative stress. They help prevent damage to blood vessels and reduce the risk of atherosclerosis, contributing to overall cardiovascular well-being.

Fiber and Heart Health

Sources:

- Whole Grains (oats, brown rice, quinoa)
- Legumes (beans, lentils)

- Fruits (apples, pears, berries)
- Vegetables (broccoli, carrots, Brussels sprouts)

Role in Heart Health:

Dietary fiber aids in maintaining healthy cholesterol levels by binding to cholesterol and promoting its excretion. It also supports blood sugar control and contributes to a healthy digestive system, indirectly benefiting heart health.

Potassium

Sources:

- Bananas
- Oranges and Orange Juice
- Potatoes (with skin)
- Spinach
- Avocado

Role in Heart Health:

Potassium helps regulate blood pressure by balancing sodium levels. Adequate potassium intake is associated with lower blood pressure, reducing the strain on the heart and lowering the risk of cardiovascular events.

Magnesium

Sources:

- Nuts and Seeds
- Whole Grains
- Leafy Green Vegetables
- Fish
- Dark Chocolate (in moderation)

Role in Heart Health:

Magnesium is crucial for maintaining a regular heart rhythm and supporting muscle function. It plays a role in dilating blood vessels, contributing to lower blood pressure and improved cardiovascular health.

Calcium

Sources:

- Dairy Products (milk, yogurt, cheese)
- Leafy Green Vegetables
- Fortified Plant-Based Milk (soy, almond)
- Tofu
- Sardines (with bones)

Role in Heart Health:

Calcium is essential for muscle function, including the heart. It contributes to blood vessel constriction and relaxation, nerve transmission, and overall cardiovascular stability.

Understanding the significance of these key nutrients and incorporating them into a well-balanced diet is instrumental in promoting heart health and reducing the risk of cardiovascular diseases, including Congestive Heart Failure.

1.2 Reading Nutritional Labels

Understanding how to decipher nutritional labels is a valuable skill in making informed and heart-healthy food choices. Nutritional labels provide essential information about the content of packaged foods, helping individuals manage their dietary intake and maintain optimal heart health. Here's a guide to reading nutritional labels effectively:

1. Serving Size:
The serving size indicates the recommended portion for the nutritional information provided. Pay attention to this, as the values listed are based on one serving.

2. Calories:
The total calories per serving are prominently displayed. Be mindful of your daily calorie needs and adjust portion sizes accordingly.

3. Macronutrients:

Total Fat:

This section breaks down fat content into saturated and trans fats. Aim for lower saturated and trans fat intake to support heart health.

Cholesterol:

Keep an eye on cholesterol levels, especially if managing cardiovascular health. Limit foods high in cholesterol for heart-friendly choices.

Sodium:

High sodium intake can contribute to hypertension. Choose products with lower sodium content, especially if you have or are at risk of high blood pressure.

Total Carbohydrates:

Pay attention to total carbohydrates and their breakdown into dietary fiber and sugars. Opt for foods higher in fiber and lower in added sugars.

Protein:

Protein is essential for overall health. Choose foods with a balance of protein, particularly if you're looking to maintain or build muscle.

4. Micronutrients:

Vitamins and Minerals:

Some labels provide information on the percentage of daily recommended intake for various vitamins and minerals. Use this as a guide to ensure a well-rounded nutrient profile.

5. Ingredients List:

Ingredients are listed in descending order by weight. Choose products with whole, recognizable ingredients, and be cautious of additives, preservatives, and excessive sugars.

6. Percent Daily Value (% DV):

This indicates how much a nutrient in a serving contributes to a daily diet. Aim for foods with a lower % DV for saturated fat, trans fat, cholesterol, and sodium, and a higher % DV for fiber, vitamins, and minerals.

7. Calories from Fat:

This provides the percentage of total calories derived from fat. It can help you assess the proportion of calories coming from fat in the product.

8. Nutrient Claims:

Pay attention to nutrient claims like "low-fat," "high-fiber," or "reduced sodium." However, always cross-verify these claims with the actual nutritional content.

9. Allergen Information:

If you have allergies or sensitivities, carefully review the allergen information to ensure the product is safe for consumption.

10. Check for Hidden Sugars:

Look for various names for added sugars (corn syrup, sucrose, high-fructose corn syrup) in the ingredients list. Be cautious of products with excessive added sugars.

Developing the habit of reading nutritional labels empowers individuals to make choices aligned with their health goals, including maintaining a heart-healthy diet. Being mindful of portion sizes and understanding the nutritional content of packaged foods contributes to overall well-being and supports cardiovascular health.

Chapter 2: Dietary Guidelines

In the pursuit of optimal heart health and the management of conditions like Congestive Heart Failure (CHF), adherence to sound dietary guidelines becomes paramount. This chapter explores comprehensive dietary recommendations, offering practical insights into crafting a nutrition plan conducive to cardiovascular well-being.

2.1 Food to Eat

In the pursuit of a heart-healthy diet and the effective management of conditions like Congestive Heart Failure (CHF), the focus on nutrient-dense and heart-supportive foods is essential. Incorporating the following foods into your daily meals can contribute to cardiovascular well-being and enhance overall health:

Fruits and Vegetables

Berries: Blueberries, strawberries, and raspberries are rich in antioxidants and vitamins.

Leafy Greens: Spinach, kale, and Swiss chard provide essential nutrients and support heart health.

Citrus Fruits: Oranges, grapefruits, lemons, and limes are excellent sources of vitamin C and fiber.

Colorful Vegetables: Bell peppers, tomatoes, carrots, and broccoli offer a spectrum of vitamins and minerals.

Whole Grains

Oats: Rich in soluble fiber, oats help manage cholesterol levels.

Quinoa: A complete protein source with fiber and various nutrients.

Brown Rice: A healthy alternative to refined grains, providing sustained energy.

Whole Wheat: Including whole wheat bread and pasta for additional fiber.

Lean Proteins

Fatty Fish: Salmon, mackerel, and trout provide omega-3 fatty acids, supporting heart health.

Skinless Poultry: Chicken and turkey are lean protein sources.

Plant-Based Proteins: Beans, lentils, tofu, and edamame offer protein with less saturated fat.

Nuts and Seeds: Almonds, walnuts, chia seeds, and flaxseeds provide healthy fats.

Healthy Fats

Olive Oil: A source of monounsaturated fats linked to heart health.

Avocados: Rich in monounsaturated fats, potassium, and fiber.

Nuts and Seeds: Almonds, walnuts, and flaxseeds contain heart-healthy fats.

Dairy or Dairy Alternatives

Low-Fat Yogurt: A source of calcium and protein without excessive saturated fat.

Skim or Low-Fat Milk: Providing calcium and vitamin D for bone health.

Plant-Based Milk Alternatives: Soy, almond, or oat milk fortified with essential nutrients.

Fiber-Rich Foods

Legumes: Beans, lentils, and chickpeas are excellent sources of fiber and protein.

Whole Fruits: Apples, pears, and berries offer natural sugars and fiber.

Vegetables: Broccoli, Brussels sprouts, and artichokes contribute to daily fiber intake.

Potassium-Rich Foods

Bananas: A potassium-rich fruit beneficial for heart health.

Oranges: Besides vitamin C, oranges provide potassium.

Potatoes (with skin): A source of potassium and dietary fiber.

Spinach: A leafy green high in potassium.

Incorporating these heart-healthy foods into your diet fosters a nutritionally rich and well-balanced approach, supporting overall cardiovascular health and assisting in the management of conditions like Congestive Heart Failure. It is advisable to personalize your diet based on individual health needs and consulting with healthcare professionals or nutrition experts for tailored advice is highly recommended.

2.2 Food to Avoid

Minimizing or avoiding the following foods can contribute to a heart-healthy lifestyle and support overall well-being:

High-Sodium Foods

Processed and Canned Foods: These often contain high levels of sodium for preservation.

Fast Food and Takeout: Restaurant meals, especially fast food, tend to be high in sodium.

Salty Snacks: Chips, pretzels, and salted nuts can contribute to excessive sodium intake.

Saturated and Trans Fats

Fried Foods: Deep-fried items such as fries and fried chicken can be high in unhealthy fats.

Fatty Cuts of Meat: Choose lean cuts and avoid excessive consumption of red or processed meats.

Full-Fat Dairy: Limit whole milk, full-fat cheeses, and creamy desserts.

Processed Foods: Many processed snacks and baked goods contain trans fats.

Added Sugars

Sugary Beverages: Sodas, sweetened juices, and energy drinks can contribute to excess sugar intake.

Candies and Sweets: Minimize the consumption of candies, cookies, and sugary desserts.

Sweetened Breakfast Cereals: Opt for whole-grain, low-sugar alternatives.

High-Caffeine and Alcoholic Beverages

Excessive Coffee and Caffeinated Drinks: While moderate coffee consumption may have benefits, excessive caffeine can lead to dehydration.

Excessive Alcohol: Limit alcohol intake, as it can contribute to dehydration and negatively impact heart function.

Processed and Refined Grains

White Bread and Pastries: Choose whole grain options for better nutritional value.

White Rice: Opt for brown rice or other whole grains for added fiber.

High-Intensity Spices and Condiments

Excessive Salt and High-Sodium Condiments: Be cautious with soy sauce, teriyaki sauce, and other condiments high in sodium.

Foods with Hidden Sodium

Canned Soups and Broths: These can be sources of hidden sodium.

Packaged Snacks: Many snack items, even those labeled as "healthy," may contain significant sodium levels.

High-Potassium Foods (for Individuals with Potassium Restrictions)

Potassium-Rich Foods: In cases where there are potassium restrictions, limit intake of high-potassium foods like bananas, oranges, and potatoes.

It's essential to note that individual dietary needs may vary, and specific recommendations should be tailored based on personal health conditions and medical advice. Consulting with healthcare professionals or nutrition experts is highly recommended to create a personalized dietary plan that aligns with individual health goals and supports the management of Congestive Heart Failure.

2.3 Adapting to Dietary Restrictions

Adapting to dietary restrictions is a crucial aspect of managing heart health, especially for individuals dealing with conditions like Congestive Heart Failure (CHF). Embracing dietary modifications tailored to specific needs can significantly contribute to overall well-being. Here are key considerations for adapting to dietary restrictions:

Sodium Restriction

Understanding Sodium Limits:

Be aware of recommended daily sodium limits and work with healthcare professionals to set individualized goals.

Mindful Food Choices:

Opt for fresh, whole foods and minimize the consumption of processed and pre-packaged items, which often contain high levels of sodium.

Smart Seasoning Alternatives:

Experiment with herbs, spices, lemon juice, and vinegar to enhance flavor without relying on excessive salt.

Fluid Management

Monitoring Fluid Intake:

Keep a fluid intake log to track daily consumption, especially if fluid restriction is advised.

Choosing Hydrating Foods:

Incorporate water-rich foods like fruits and vegetables to contribute to hydration without solely relying on beverages.

Adjusting Based on Individual Needs:

Work closely with healthcare professionals to determine personalized fluid intake goals based on specific health conditions.

Potassium Management

Understanding Potassium Limits:

Be aware of recommended potassium limits, particularly if there are restrictions due to medications or kidney issues.

Identifying High-Potassium Foods:

Learn to identify and limit high-potassium foods, such as bananas, oranges, and certain vegetables.

Balancing Nutrient Intake:

Focus on a well-balanced diet, incorporating a variety of foods to ensure adequate nutrition while managing potassium levels.

Nutrient-Dense Substitutions

Healthy Fat Alternatives:

Choose sources of healthy fats, such as avocados, nuts, and olive oil, as substitutes for saturated and trans fats.

Lean Protein Options:

Opt for lean protein sources like fish, poultry, tofu, and legumes while minimizing red and processed meats.

Whole Grain Choices:

Replace refined grains with whole grains like brown rice, quinoa, and whole wheat for added fiber and nutrients.

Individualized Meal Planning

Consulting with Nutrition Professionals:

Seek guidance from dietitians or nutritionists to create personalized meal plans aligned with dietary restrictions.

Adapting Recipes:

Modify recipes to meet specific needs, adjusting ingredients and portion sizes as necessary.

Supportive Community Engagement:

Connect with support groups or communities to share experiences, recipes, and tips for adapting to dietary restrictions.

Education and Empowerment

Continuous Learning:

Stay informed about dietary guidelines, potential challenges, and new approaches to managing dietary restrictions.

Advocating for Health Needs:

Be an advocate for your health by actively participating in discussions with healthcare professionals and making informed choices.

Adapting to dietary restrictions is a dynamic and ongoing process. With a proactive approach, collaboration with healthcare professionals, and a commitment to making informed food choices, individuals can successfully navigate and embrace a heart-healthy lifestyle tailored to their specific needs and conditions.

Chapter 3: Breakfast Boosters

Berry Power Smoothie Bowl

Preparation Time: 10 minutes

Servings: 2

Ingredients:

- 1 cup mixed berries (strawberries, blueberries, raspberries)
- 1 ripe banana, frozen
- 1/2 cup low-fat Greek yogurt
- 1/4 cup almond milk (or any preferred milk)
- 1 tablespoon chia seeds
- 1 tablespoon honey or maple syrup (optional, for sweetness)
- Toppings: Fresh berries, sliced almonds, granola

Preparation:

1. Wash the berries thoroughly and set aside a handful for topping. Keep a mix of berries for a vibrant flavor profile.
2. Peel and slice the ripe banana before freezing it. The frozen banana adds a creamy texture to the smoothie bowl.
3. In a blender, combine the mixed berries, frozen banana slices, low-fat Greek yogurt, almond milk, chia seeds, and sweetener if desired. Blend until you achieve a smooth and creamy consistency.

4. Pour the smoothie into a bowl. The thickness should be similar to that of soft-serve ice cream.

5. Top your smoothie bowl with the reserved fresh berries, sliced almonds, and a sprinkle of granola for added crunch and nutrition.

6. If you have a sweet tooth, drizzle honey or maple syrup over the top for that extra touch of sweetness.

Avocado Toast with Poached Egg

Preparation Time: 15 minutes

Servings: 2

Ingredients:

- 2 slices whole-grain bread
- 1 ripe avocado
- 2 large eggs
- Salt and pepper to taste
- Optional toppings: Red pepper flakes, cherry tomatoes, feta cheese

Preparation:

1. Toast the slices of whole-grain bread to your desired level of crispiness.

2. Mash the ripe avocado and spread it evenly on the toasted bread slices.

3. Poach the eggs until the whites are set but the yolks are still runny. If you're not familiar with poaching, you can also opt for fried or boiled eggs.

4. Carefully place the poached eggs on top of the mashed avocado.

5. Season with salt and pepper to taste. Add optional toppings like red pepper flakes, halved cherry tomatoes, or crumbled feta cheese for extra flavor.

6. Serve the avocado toast with poached egg immediately while it's warm. The combination of creamy avocado and a perfectly poached egg creates a satisfying and nutritious breakfast.

Quinoa Breakfast Bowl

Preparation Time: 20 minutes

Servings: 2

Ingredients:

- 1 cup cooked quinoa
- 1/2 cup almond milk (or any preferred milk)
- 1 tablespoon honey or maple syrup
- 1/2 teaspoon vanilla extract
- Toppings: Sliced bananas, chopped nuts, dried fruits, a sprinkle of cinnamon

Preparation:

1. Cook quinoa according to package instructions. Fluff it with a fork once cooked.

2. In a bowl, combine the cooked quinoa, almond milk, honey or maple syrup, and vanilla extract. Mix well to create a creamy base.

3. Divide the quinoa mixture into bowls.

4. Top the quinoa with sliced bananas, chopped nuts, dried fruits, and a sprinkle of cinnamon.

5. This quinoa breakfast bowl is a nutrient-rich and satisfying option to fuel your day. Enjoy the wholesome combination of grains, fruits, and nuts in every spoonful.

Greek Yogurt Parfait

Preparation Time: 10 minutes

Servings: 2

Ingredients:
- 1 cup Greek yogurt
- 1/2 cup granola
- 1/2 cup mixed berries (strawberries, blueberries, raspberries)
- Honey for drizzling

Preparation:
1. In serving glasses or bowls, start by layering Greek yogurt at the bottom.

2. Sprinkle a layer of granola over the Greek yogurt.

3. Add a layer of mixed berries on top of the granola.

4. Repeat the layers until the glass or bowl is filled, finishing with a generous layer of berries on top.

5. Drizzle honey over the parfait for a touch of sweetness.

6. Refrigerate the parfaits for a while before serving. The cool and creamy layers combined with the crunch of granola create a delightful and nutritious breakfast or snack.

Spinach and Feta Omelette

Preparation Time: 15 minutes

Servings: 2

Ingredients:

- 4 large eggs
- 1 cup fresh spinach, chopped
- 1/2 cup feta cheese, crumbled
- 1/4 cup red bell pepper, diced
- 1/4 cup red onion, finely chopped
- Salt and pepper to taste
- Olive oil for cooking

Preparation:

1. In a bowl, whisk the eggs until well combined. Season with salt and pepper.
2. In a non-stick skillet, heat olive oil over medium heat. Sauté the chopped spinach, red bell pepper, and red onion until the vegetables are softened.
3. Pour the whisked eggs over the sautéed vegetables in the skillet.
4. Sprinkle crumbled feta cheese evenly over the eggs.
5. Allow the omelet to cook without stirring until the edges are set. Then, gently lift the edges with a spatula to let any uncooked eggs flow underneath.
6. Once the eggs are mostly set but slightly runny on top, fold the omelet in half. Continue cooking until the eggs are fully set but still moist inside.
7. Slide the omelet onto a plate and serve it warm. This spinach and feta omelet is a delicious and protein-packed breakfast option.

Chia Seed Pudding

Preparation Time: 5 minutes (plus chilling time)

Servings: 2

Ingredients:
- 1/4 cup chia seeds
- 1 cup almond milk (or any preferred milk)
- 1 tablespoon maple syrup or honey

- 1/2 teaspoon vanilla extract
- Fresh berries for topping

Preparation:

1. In a bowl, whisk together chia seeds, almond milk, maple syrup (or honey), and vanilla extract.
2. Cover the bowl and refrigerate for at least 2 hours or overnight to allow the chia seeds to absorb the liquid and form a pudding-like consistency.
3. Before serving, give the pudding a good stir. If it's too thick, you can add a bit more almond milk to reach your desired consistency.
4. Top with fresh berries and enjoy this nutritious and satisfying chia seed pudding.

Banana Nut Oatmeal

Preparation Time: 10 minutes

Servings: 2

Ingredients:

- 1 cup old-fashioned oats
- 2 cups water or milk
- 1 ripe banana, mashed
- 1/4 cup chopped nuts (walnuts, almonds, or pecans)
- 1 tablespoon honey or maple syrup

- Dash of cinnamon
- Sliced banana for garnish (optional)

Preparation:

1. In a saucepan, bring water or milk to a boil.
2. Stir in the old-fashioned oats and reduce the heat to medium-low. Cook, stirring occasionally, until the oats are creamy and cooked to your liking.
3. Mix in the mashed banana, chopped nuts, honey (or maple syrup), and a dash of cinnamon.
4. Continue cooking for an additional 2-3 minutes until the banana is well incorporated and the oats are thoroughly cooked.
5. Serve the banana nut oatmeal warm, garnished with sliced banana if desired. This wholesome breakfast is both comforting and nutritious.

Cottage Cheese and Pineapple Bowl

Preparation Time: 5 minutes

Servings: 1

Ingredients:

- 1 cup cottage cheese
- 1/2 cup fresh pineapple chunks
- 1 tablespoon honey
- Optional: Chopped mint for garnish

Preparation:

1. In a bowl, combine cottage cheese and fresh pineapple chunks.

2. Drizzle honey over the mixture.

3. Gently toss to coat the cottage cheese and pineapple with honey.

4. Garnish with chopped mint if desired.

5. Enjoy this quick and protein-packed cottage cheese and pineapple bowl for a refreshing breakfast.

Sweet Potato Breakfast Hash

Preparation Time: 20 minutes

Servings: 2

Ingredients:

- 2 medium sweet potatoes, peeled and diced
- 1 tablespoon olive oil
- 1/2 onion, diced
- 1 bell pepper, diced
- 1 cup spinach, chopped
- 2 eggs (optional)
- Salt and pepper to taste
- Paprika and cumin for seasoning

Preparation:

1. In a skillet, heat olive oil over medium heat.

2. Add diced sweet potatoes and cook until they start to brown and become tender.

3. Add diced onion and bell pepper to the skillet. Cook until the vegetables are softened.

4. Stir in chopped spinach and season with salt, pepper, paprika, and cumin. Cook until the spinach wilts.

5. If desired, create wells in the hash and crack eggs into them. Cover the skillet and cook until the eggs are cooked to your liking.

6. Serve the sweet potato breakfast hash warm, adjusting seasoning if needed. This hearty and flavorful dish is a great way to start your day.

Blueberry Almond Overnight Oats

Preparation Time: 5 minutes (plus chilling time)

Servings: 2

Ingredients:
- 1 cup old-fashioned oats
- 1 cup almond milk (or any preferred milk)
- 1/2 cup fresh blueberries
- 2 tablespoons almond butter
- 1 tablespoon honey or maple syrup
- 1/4 teaspoon almond extract (optional)
- Sliced almonds for topping

Preparation:

1. In a jar or container, combine old-fashioned oats, almond milk, fresh blueberries, almond butter, honey (or maple syrup), and almond extract if using.

2. Stir well to ensure all ingredients are evenly distributed.

3. Cover the jar or container and refrigerate overnight or for at least 4 hours.

4. Before serving, give the overnight oats a good stir. If the consistency is too thick, you can add a bit more almond milk.

5. Top with sliced almonds and enjoy these delicious and convenient blueberry almond overnight oats.

Egg White Veggie Scramble

Preparation Time: 15 minutes

Servings: 2

Ingredients:

- 4 egg whites
- 1 tablespoon olive oil
- 1/2 onion, diced
- 1 bell pepper, diced
- 1 cup spinach, chopped
- Salt and pepper to taste
- Optional: Feta cheese for garnish

Preparation:

1. In a bowl, whisk the egg whites until frothy.
2. In a skillet, heat olive oil over medium heat.
3. Add diced onion and bell pepper to the skillet. Cook until the vegetables are softened.
4. Add chopped spinach to the skillet and cook until wilted.
5. Pour the whisked egg whites over the vegetables. Season with salt and pepper.
6. Gently scramble the eggs until fully cooked.
7. If desired, garnish with crumbled feta cheese.
8. Serve the egg white veggie scramble warm. This protein-packed breakfast is light, flavorful, and full of nutritious veggies.

Apple Cinnamon Quinoa Porridge

Preparation Time: 20 minutes

Servings: 2

Ingredients:

- 1/2 cup quinoa, rinsed
- 1 cup water
- 1 cup milk (dairy or plant-based)
- 1 apple, peeled, cored, and diced
- 1 tablespoon maple syrup or honey

- 1/2 teaspoon ground cinnamon
- 1/4 cup chopped nuts (walnuts or almonds)
- Optional: Greek yogurt for topping

Preparation:

1. In a saucepan, combine quinoa and water. Bring to a boil, then reduce heat, cover, and simmer for 15 minutes or until quinoa is cooked and water is absorbed.
2. In a separate saucepan, heat the milk over medium heat until warm.
3. Add the cooked quinoa to the warm milk, stirring to combine.
4. Stir in diced apple, maple syrup (or honey), and ground cinnamon. Cook for an additional 5 minutes, allowing the flavors to meld.
5. Remove from heat and let it sit for a few minutes to thicken.
6. Serve the apple cinnamon quinoa porridge in bowls, topped with chopped nuts and a dollop of Greek yogurt if desired. Enjoy this hearty and flavorful breakfast.

Smoked Salmon and Cream Cheese Bagel

Preparation Time: 10 minutes

Servings: 2

Ingredients:

- 2 whole-grain bagels, sliced and toasted
- 4 oz smoked salmon

- 4 tablespoons cream cheese
- Red onion, thinly sliced
- Capers for garnish
- Fresh dill for garnish
- Lemon wedges

Preparation:

1. Spread cream cheese evenly on each half of the toasted bagels.
2. Layer smoked salmon on top of the cream cheese.
3. Add thinly sliced red onion rings to the salmon.
4. Garnish with capers and fresh dill.
5. Squeeze lemon wedges over the smoked salmon and cream cheese bagels.
6. Serve immediately and savor the delightful combination of flavors in this classic breakfast option.

Mango Coconut Chia Smoothie

Preparation Time: 10 minutes (plus chilling time)

Servings: 2

Ingredients:

- 1 cup mango chunks (fresh or frozen)
- 1 cup coconut milk
- 2 tablespoons chia seeds

- 1 tablespoon honey or agave syrup
- 1/2 teaspoon vanilla extract
- Ice cubes (optional)

Preparation:

1. In a blender, combine mango chunks, coconut milk, chia seeds, honey (or agave syrup), and vanilla extract.
2. Blend until smooth and well combined.
3. Refrigerate the smoothie for at least 1 hour to allow the chia seeds to expand and create a thicker texture.
4. Before serving, give the smoothie a good stir. If it's too thick, you can add a bit more coconut milk.
5. Pour into glasses over ice cubes if desired. This mango coconut chia smoothie is a refreshing and nutrient-packed way to start your day.

Peanut Butter Banana Protein Pancakes

Preparation Time: 15 minutes

Servings: 2-3

Ingredients:

- 1 cup pancake mix
- 1/2 cup milk (dairy or plant-based)
- 1 ripe banana, mashed
- 2 tablespoons peanut butter

- 1 egg
- 1 scoop protein powder (vanilla or chocolate)
- Butter or oil for cooking
- Sliced bananas and a drizzle of peanut butter for topping

Preparation:

1. In a mixing bowl, combine pancake mix, milk, mashed banana, peanut butter, egg, and protein powder. Mix until well combined.
2. Heat a griddle or non-stick skillet over medium heat. Add a small amount of butter or oil to coat the surface.
3. Pour 1/4 cup portions of batter onto the griddle to form pancakes.
4. Cook until bubbles form on the surface, then flip and cook the other side until golden brown.
5. Repeat until all the batter is used.
6. Serve the peanut butter banana protein pancakes topped with sliced bananas and a drizzle of peanut butter. These pancakes are a delicious and protein-rich twist on a classic breakfast favorite.

Chapter 4: Luscious Lunches

Mediterranean Quinoa Salad

Preparation Time: 15 minutes

Servings: 4

Ingredients:

- 1 cup quinoa, cooked and cooled
- 1 cup cherry tomatoes, halved
- 1 cucumber, diced
- 1/2 cup Kalamata olives, sliced
- 1/2 cup red onion, finely chopped
- 1/2 cup feta cheese, crumbled
- 1/4 cup fresh parsley, chopped
- 2 tablespoons olive oil
- 1 tablespoon red wine vinegar
- Salt and pepper to taste
- Lemon wedges for serving

Preparation:

1. In a large bowl, combine cooked quinoa, cherry tomatoes, cucumber, Kalamata olives, red onion, feta cheese, and fresh parsley.

2. In a small bowl, whisk together olive oil and red wine vinegar. Pour over the quinoa mixture and toss to coat.

3. Season with salt and pepper to taste.

4. Chill in the refrigerator for at least 30 minutes before serving.

5. Serve the Mediterranean quinoa salad with lemon wedges on the side for an extra burst of flavor.

Grilled Chicken and Avocado Wrap

Preparation Time: 20 minutes

Servings: 2

Ingredients:

- 2 boneless, skinless chicken breasts
- 2 tablespoons olive oil
- 1 teaspoon smoked paprika
- 1 teaspoon garlic powder
- Salt and pepper to taste
- 2 whole-grain wraps or tortillas
- 1 avocado, sliced
- 1 cup mixed greens (spinach, arugula, or lettuce)
- 1/2 cup cherry tomatoes, halved
- Greek yogurt or tzatziki for drizzling

Preparation:

1. Preheat the grill or grill pan over medium-high heat.

2. In a bowl, mix olive oil, smoked paprika, garlic powder, salt, and pepper. Coat the chicken breasts with the mixture.

3. Grill the chicken for about 6-8 minutes per side or until fully cooked.

4. Slice the grilled chicken into strips.

5. Warm the wraps or tortillas according to package instructions.

6. Assemble the wraps by placing sliced avocado, mixed greens, cherry tomatoes, and grilled chicken on each wrap.

7. Drizzle with Greek yogurt or tzatziki.

8. Fold the wraps and secure them with toothpicks if needed.

9. Serve the grilled chicken and avocado wraps immediately.

Vegetarian Buddha Bowl with Tahini Dressing

Preparation Time: 25 minutes

Servings: 2

Ingredients:
- 1 cup quinoa, cooked
- 1 cup chickpeas, cooked or canned
- 1 cup broccoli florets, steamed
- 1 carrot, julienned
- 1/2 avocado, sliced
- 1/2 cup red cabbage, shredded
- 2 tablespoons sesame seeds, toasted

- Fresh cilantro for garnish

Tahini Dressing:

- 3 tablespoons tahini
- 2 tablespoons water
- 1 tablespoon lemon juice
- 1 clove garlic, minced
- Salt and pepper to taste

Preparation:

1. Assemble the Buddha bowls by arranging cooked quinoa, chickpeas, steamed broccoli, julienned carrot, sliced avocado, shredded red cabbage, and toasted sesame seeds in a bowl.
2. In a small bowl, whisk together tahini, water, lemon juice, minced garlic, salt, and pepper to create the dressing.
3. Drizzle the tahini dressing over the Buddha bowls.
4. Garnish with fresh cilantro.
5. Serve the vegetarian Buddha bowl with tahini dressing and enjoy a wholesome and colorful meal.

Salmon and Asparagus Foil Pack

Preparation Time: 25 minutes

Servings: 2

Ingredients:

- 2 salmon fillets
- 1 bunch asparagus, trimmed
- 2 tablespoons olive oil
- 2 cloves garlic, minced
- 1 lemon, thinly sliced
- 1 teaspoon dried dill
- Salt and pepper to taste

Preparation:

1. Preheat the oven to 400°F (200°C).
2. Place each salmon fillet in the center of a large piece of aluminum foil.
3. Arrange asparagus around the salmon fillets.
4. Drizzle olive oil over the salmon and asparagus. Sprinkle minced garlic, dried dill, salt, and pepper.
5. Place lemon slices on top of each salmon fillet.
6. Fold the foil to create a sealed packet.
7. Bake in the preheated oven for 20 minutes or until the salmon is cooked through and flakes easily.
8. Carefully open the foil packets, and transfer the salmon and asparagus to plates.
9. Serve the salmon and asparagus foil pack with additional lemon slices if desired.

Caprese Stuffed Portobello Mushrooms

Preparation Time: 30 minutes

Servings: 2

Ingredients:

- 4 large Portobello mushrooms, stems removed
- 1 cup cherry tomatoes, halved
- 1 cup fresh mozzarella, diced
- 1/4 cup fresh basil, chopped
- 2 tablespoons balsamic glaze
- 2 tablespoons olive oil
- Salt and pepper to taste

Preparation:

1. Preheat the oven to 375°F (190°C).
2. Place the Portobello mushrooms on a baking sheet.
3. In a bowl, mix cherry tomatoes, fresh mozzarella, fresh basil, olive oil, salt, and pepper.
4. Stuff each Portobello mushroom with the tomato and mozzarella mixture.
5. Bake in the preheated oven for 20 minutes or until the mushrooms are tender and the cheese is melted.
6. Drizzle with balsamic glaze before serving.
7. Serve the Caprese stuffed Portobello mushrooms as a delightful and flavorful dish.

Chickpea and Spinach Curry

Preparation Time: 30 minutes

Servings: 4

Ingredients:

- 2 tablespoons coconut oil
- 1 onion, finely chopped
- 3 cloves garlic, minced
- 1 tablespoon ginger, grated
- 1 tablespoon curry powder
- 1 teaspoon ground cumin
- 1 teaspoon ground coriander
- 1/2 teaspoon turmeric
- 1/2 teaspoon chili powder (adjust to taste)
- 1 can (15 oz) chickpeas, drained and rinsed
- 1 can (14 oz) diced tomatoes
- 1 can (14 oz) coconut milk
- 4 cups fresh spinach
- Salt and pepper to taste
- Cooked rice for serving

Preparation:

1. In a large pan, heat coconut oil over medium heat.
2. Add chopped onion and sauté until softened.

3. Stir in minced garlic and grated ginger, cooking for an additional minute.

4. Add curry powder, ground cumin, ground coriander, turmeric, and chili powder. Stir well to combine the spices with the aromatics.

5. Pour in chickpeas, diced tomatoes (with their juice), and coconut milk. Bring to a simmer and let it cook for about 15 minutes.

6. Add fresh spinach to the pan and cook until wilted.

7. Season with salt and pepper to taste.

8. Serve the chickpea and spinach curry over cooked rice for a delicious and nutritious vegetarian meal.

Turkey and Hummus Collard Green Wraps

Preparation Time: 15 minutes

Servings: 2

Ingredients:

- 4 large collard green leaves, stems removed
- 1/2 pound thinly sliced turkey breast
- 1/2 cup hummus
- 1 cucumber, julienned
- 1 carrot, julienned
- 1 red bell pepper, thinly sliced
- Fresh herbs (such as cilantro or mint) for garnish
- Salt and pepper to taste

Preparation:

1. Blanch collard green leaves in boiling water for 30 seconds. Transfer to an ice bath to cool.
2. Lay the collard green leaves flat on a clean surface.
3. Spread hummus evenly over each collard green leaf.
4. Layer sliced turkey, julienned cucumber, carrot, and red bell pepper on each leaf.
5. Season with salt and pepper to taste.
6. Fold in the sides of the collard green leaves and roll them up tightly to form wraps.
7. Secure with toothpicks if needed.
8. Garnish with fresh herbs and serve the turkey and hummus collard green wraps.

Sweet Potato and Black Bean Quesadillas

Preparation Time: 30 minutes

Servings: 2

Ingredients:

- 2 large whole-grain tortillas
- 1 large sweet potato, cooked and mashed
- 1 cup black beans, cooked or canned, drained and rinsed
- 1 cup shredded cheddar cheese

- 1 teaspoon ground cumin
- 1/2 teaspoon chili powder
- 1/2 teaspoon garlic powder
- Salt and pepper to taste
- Olive oil for cooking

Preparation:

1. In a bowl, mix mashed sweet potato, black beans, ground cumin, chili powder, garlic powder, salt, and pepper.
2. Place a tortilla on a flat surface.
3. Spread half of the sweet potato and black bean mixture evenly over one-half of the tortilla.
4. Sprinkle half of the shredded cheddar cheese over the sweet potato mixture.
5. Fold the other half of the tortilla over the filling to create a half-moon shape.
6. Repeat the process for the second quesadilla.
7. Heat olive oil in a skillet over medium heat.
8. Cook each quesadilla for 3-4 minutes on each side or until the tortilla is golden and the cheese is melted.
9. Slice and serve the sweet potato and black bean quesadillas with your favorite salsa or guacamole.

Cauliflower Fried Rice with Shrimp

Preparation Time: 25 minutes

Servings: 2

Ingredients:

- 1 small cauliflower, grated or riced
- 1/2 pound shrimp, peeled and deveined
- 1 cup mixed vegetables (peas, carrots, corn)
- 2 eggs, beaten
- 3 tablespoons soy sauce
- 2 tablespoons sesame oil
- 2 green onions, chopped
- 1 clove garlic, minced
- 1 teaspoon ginger, grated
- Salt and pepper to taste

Preparation:

1. Heat sesame oil in a large skillet over medium heat.
2. Add shrimp and cook until they turn pink. Remove from the skillet and set aside.
3. In the same skillet, add garlic and ginger. Sauté for 1-2 minutes until fragrant.
4. Add mixed vegetables to the skillet and cook until they are tender-crisp.
5. Push the vegetables to one side of the skillet and pour the beaten eggs into the empty side. Scramble the eggs until cooked through.

6. Add grated cauliflower to the skillet, along with soy sauce and cooked shrimp. Stir well to combine.

7. Cook for an additional 5-7 minutes, allowing the cauliflower to cook and absorb the flavors.

8. Season with salt and pepper to taste.

9. Garnish with chopped green onions and serve the cauliflower fried rice with shrimp.

Mango Avocado Chicken Salad

Preparation Time: 20 minutes

Servings: 2

Ingredients:

- 2 boneless, skinless chicken breasts, cooked and shredded
- 1 mango, peeled and diced
- 1 avocado, peeled and diced
- 1/2 red onion, finely chopped
- 1/4 cup cilantro, chopped
- Juice of 1 lime
- 2 tablespoons olive oil
- Salt and pepper to taste
- Mixed salad greens for serving

Preparation:

In a large bowl, combine shredded chicken, diced mango, diced avocado, chopped red onion, and cilantro.

In a small bowl, whisk together lime juice, olive oil, salt, and pepper.

Pour the dressing over the chicken mixture and toss to coat evenly.

Serve the mango avocado chicken salad over a bed of mixed salad greens.

Tomato Basil Mozzarella Panini

Preparation Time: 15 minutes

Servings: 2

Ingredients:
- 4 slices whole-grain bread
- 1 large tomato, thinly sliced
- Fresh mozzarella cheese, sliced
- Fresh basil leaves
- Olive oil for brushing
- Balsamic glaze for drizzling (optional)
- Salt and pepper to taste

Preparation:
1. Preheat a panini press or a skillet over medium heat.
2. Place tomato slices, fresh mozzarella slices, and basil leaves on two slices of bread.

3. Season with salt and pepper to taste.

4. Top with the remaining slices of bread.

5. Brush the outside of each sandwich with olive oil.

6. Grill the panini in the press or skillet until the bread is golden and the cheese is melted.

7. Drizzle with balsamic glaze if desired.

8. Slice and serve the tomato basil mozzarella panini.

Lentil and Vegetable Soup

Preparation Time: 40 minutes

Servings: 4

Ingredients:

- 1 cup dried green or brown lentils, rinsed
- 1 onion, chopped
- 2 carrots, diced
- 2 celery stalks, diced
- 3 cloves garlic, minced
- 1 can (14 oz) diced tomatoes
- 6 cups vegetable broth
- 1 teaspoon ground cumin
- 1 teaspoon ground coriander
- 1/2 teaspoon smoked paprika
- Salt and pepper to taste

- Fresh parsley for garnish

Preparation:

1. In a large pot, sauté chopped onion, diced carrots, and diced celery until softened.
2. Add minced garlic and cook for an additional 1-2 minutes.
3. Stir in dried lentils, diced tomatoes, vegetable broth, ground cumin, ground coriander, smoked paprika, salt, and pepper.
4. Bring the soup to a boil, then reduce heat and simmer for 25-30 minutes or until lentils are tender.
5. Adjust seasoning if needed.
6. Garnish with fresh parsley before serving the lentil and vegetable soup.

Quinoa and Roasted Vegetable Stuffed Peppers

Preparation Time: 40 minutes

Servings: 4

Ingredients:

- 4 large bell peppers, halved and seeds removed
- 1 cup quinoa, cooked
- 2 cups mixed roasted vegetables (zucchini, bell peppers, cherry tomatoes, etc.)
- 1 cup black beans, cooked or canned, drained and rinsed

- 1 cup corn kernels (fresh or frozen)
- 1 cup shredded cheese (cheddar, Monterey Jack, or your choice)
- 1 teaspoon ground cumin
- 1 teaspoon chili powder
- 1/2 teaspoon garlic powder
- Salt and pepper to taste
- Fresh cilantro or parsley for garnish
- Olive oil for drizzling

Preparation:

1. Preheat the oven to 375°F (190°C).
2. Place the halved bell peppers in a baking dish.
3. In a large bowl, combine cooked quinoa, roasted vegetables, black beans, corn, shredded cheese, ground cumin, chili powder, garlic powder, salt, and pepper. Mix well.
4. Stuff each bell pepper half with the quinoa and roasted vegetable mixture.
5. Drizzle olive oil over the stuffed peppers.
6. Bake in the preheated oven for 25-30 minutes or until the peppers are tender and the filling is heated through.
7. Garnish with fresh cilantro or parsley before serving.

Asian Sesame Ginger Tofu Bowl

Preparation Time: 30 minutes

Servings: 2

Ingredients:

- 1 cup tofu, cubed
- 2 tablespoons soy sauce
- 1 tablespoon sesame oil
- 1 tablespoon rice vinegar
- 1 tablespoon honey or agave syrup
- 1 teaspoon grated ginger
- 2 cloves garlic, minced
- 1 cup broccoli florets
- 1 carrot, julienned
- 1 bell pepper, thinly sliced
- 2 cups cooked brown rice
- Sesame seeds and green onions for garnish

Preparation:

1. In a bowl, marinate tofu cubes in soy sauce, sesame oil, rice vinegar, honey, grated ginger, and minced garlic. Let it marinate for at least 15 minutes.
2. In a skillet, sauté marinated tofu until golden and crispy on the edges.
3. In the same skillet, stir-fry broccoli, julienned carrot, and sliced bell pepper until they are tender-crisp.
4. Serve the sautéed tofu and vegetables over cooked brown rice.
5. Garnish with sesame seeds and chopped green onions before serving.

Pesto Zucchini Noodles with Cherry Tomatoes

Preparation Time: 20 minutes

Servings: 2

Ingredients:

- 3 medium zucchini, spiralized into noodles
- 1 cup cherry tomatoes, halved
- 1/2 cup fresh basil leaves
- 1/4 cup pine nuts
- 1/4 cup grated Parmesan cheese
- 2 cloves garlic
- 1/3 cup extra virgin olive oil
- Salt and pepper to taste
- Red pepper flakes for a hint of spice (optional)

Preparation:

1. In a food processor, combine fresh basil, pine nuts, grated Parmesan, and garlic. Pulse until coarsely chopped.
2. With the food processor running, slowly add the olive oil until the pesto reaches a smooth consistency.
3. Season the pesto with salt and pepper to taste. Add red pepper flakes if you desire some heat.
4. In a large skillet, heat a bit of olive oil over medium heat.

5. Add zucchini noodles and cherry tomatoes to the skillet. Sauté for 2-3 minutes until the noodles are just tender.

6. Toss the zucchini noodles and cherry tomatoes with the prepared pesto until evenly coated.

7. Serve the pesto zucchini noodles with cherry tomatoes, garnished with additional Parmesan if desired.

Chapter 5: Delectable Dinners

Lemon Garlic Roasted Chicken with Rosemary Potatoes

Preparation Time: 1 hour

Servings: 4

Ingredients:

- 4 bone-in, skin-on chicken thighs
- 1.5 lbs baby potatoes, halved
- 4 cloves garlic, minced
- 1 lemon, zest, and juice
- 2 tablespoons olive oil
- 1 tablespoon fresh rosemary, chopped
- Salt and pepper to taste

Preparation:

1. Preheat the oven to 400°F (200°C).
2. In a bowl, mix minced garlic, lemon zest, lemon juice, olive oil, chopped rosemary, salt, and pepper.
3. Place chicken thighs and halved baby potatoes on a baking sheet.
4. Brush the chicken and potatoes with the lemon garlic mixture, ensuring they are well-coated.

5. Roast in the preheated oven for about 40-45 minutes or until the chicken is golden brown and cooked through, and the potatoes are tender.

6. Serve the lemon garlic roasted chicken with rosemary potatoes.

Shrimp and Quinoa Stuffed Bell Peppers

Preparation Time: 40 minutes

Servings: 4

Ingredients:

- 4 bell peppers, halved and seeds removed
- 1 cup quinoa, cooked
- 1 lb shrimp, peeled and deveined, chopped
- 1 cup black beans, cooked or canned, drained and rinsed
- 1 cup corn kernels (fresh or frozen)
- 1 cup diced tomatoes
- 1 teaspoon cumin
- 1 teaspoon chili powder
- 1/2 teaspoon garlic powder
- Salt and pepper to taste
- 1 cup shredded cheese (cheddar or Monterey Jack)
- Fresh cilantro for garnish

Preparation

1. Preheat the oven to 375°F (190°C).

2. Place bell pepper halves in a baking dish.

3. In a bowl, combine cooked quinoa, chopped shrimp, black beans, corn, diced tomatoes, cumin, chili powder, garlic powder, salt, and pepper.

4. Stuff each bell pepper half with the quinoa and shrimp mixture.

5. Top each stuffed pepper with shredded cheese.

6. Bake in the preheated oven for 25-30 minutes or until the peppers are tender, and the cheese is melted and bubbly.

7. Garnish with fresh cilantro before serving.

Vegetarian Chickpea Tikka Masala

Preparation Time: 35 minutes

Servings: 4

Ingredients:

- 2 cans (15 oz each) chickpeas, drained and rinsed
- 1 large onion, finely chopped
- 3 cloves garlic, minced
- 1 tablespoon ginger, grated
- 1 can (14 oz) diced tomatoes
- 1/2 cup tomato sauce
- 1/2 cup plain yogurt
- 2 teaspoons garam masala

- 1 teaspoon ground cumin
- 1 teaspoon ground coriander
- 1/2 teaspoon turmeric
- 1/2 teaspoon paprika
- Salt and pepper to taste
- Fresh cilantro for garnish
- Cooked rice for serving

Preparation:

1. In a large pan, sauté chopped onion until softened.
2. Add minced garlic and grated ginger, cooking for an additional 1-2 minutes.
3. Stir in garam masala, ground cumin, ground coriander, turmeric, paprika, salt, and pepper.
4. Add chickpeas, diced tomatoes (with their juice), and tomato sauce to the pan. Simmer for 15-20 minutes.
5. Stir in plain yogurt and cook for an additional 5 minutes.
6. Adjust seasoning if needed.
7. Serve the vegetarian chickpea tikka masala over cooked rice, garnished with fresh cilantro.

Grilled Salmon with Dill Yogurt Sauce

Preparation Time: 20 minutes

Servings: 2

Ingredients:

- 2 salmon fillets
- 2 tablespoons olive oil
- 1 teaspoon lemon zest
- 1 tablespoon lemon juice
- 1 teaspoon Dijon mustard
- 1 tablespoon fresh dill, chopped
- Salt and pepper to taste

Dill Yogurt Sauce:

- 1/2 cup Greek yogurt
- 1 tablespoon fresh dill, chopped
- 1 teaspoon lemon juice
- Salt and pepper to taste

Preparation:

1. Preheat the grill or grill pan over medium-high heat.
2. In a bowl, mix olive oil, lemon zest, lemon juice, Dijon mustard, chopped dill, salt, and pepper.
3. Brush the salmon fillets with the lemon dill mixture.
4. Grill the salmon for about 4-5 minutes per side or until cooked to your liking.
5. In a small bowl, whisk together Greek yogurt, chopped dill, lemon juice, salt, and pepper to make the dill yogurt sauce.
6. Serve the grilled salmon with a dollop of dill yogurt sauce.

Eggplant Parmesan with Whole Wheat Pasta

Preparation Time: 1 hour

Servings: 4

Ingredients:

- 1 large eggplant, sliced into rounds
- 2 cups whole wheat pasta, cooked
- 2 cups marinara sauce
- 1 cup mozzarella cheese, shredded
- 1/2 cup Parmesan cheese, grated
- 1/4 cup fresh basil, chopped
- 2 tablespoons olive oil
- Salt and pepper to taste

Preparation:

1. Preheat the oven to 375°F (190°C).
2. Brush eggplant slices with olive oil and season with salt and pepper.
3. Roast the eggplant slices in the oven for 20-25 minutes or until they are tender.
4. In a baking dish, layer cooked whole wheat pasta, marinara sauce, roasted eggplant slices, mozzarella cheese, and Parmesan cheese.
5. Repeat the layers, finishing with a layer of cheese on top.
6. Bake in the preheated oven for 20-25 minutes or until the cheese is melted and bubbly.

7. Garnish with chopped fresh basil before serving.

Teriyaki Tofu Stir-Fry with Broccoli and Bell Peppers

Preparation Time: 30 minutes

Servings: 4

Ingredients:

- 1 block extra-firm tofu, pressed and cubed
- 2 cups broccoli florets
- 1 red bell pepper, sliced
- 1 yellow bell pepper, sliced
- 1 carrot, julienned
- 1/2 cup teriyaki sauce
- 2 tablespoons soy sauce
- 1 tablespoon sesame oil
- 1 tablespoon cornstarch
- 2 tablespoons vegetable oil for stir-frying
- Cooked brown rice for serving
- Sesame seeds and green onions for garnish

Preparation:

1. In a bowl, mix teriyaki sauce, soy sauce, sesame oil, and cornstarch to create the sauce.
2. Heat vegetable oil in a large wok or skillet over medium-high heat.

3. Add cubed tofu and stir-fry until golden and crispy.

4. Remove tofu from the wok and set aside.

5. In the same wok, add more oil if needed, and stir-fry broccoli, red bell pepper, yellow bell pepper, and julienned carrot until they are tender-crisp.

6. Add the cooked tofu back to the wok and pour the teriyaki sauce over the tofu and vegetables.

7. Toss everything together until well coated and heated through.

8. Serve the teriyaki tofu stir-fry over cooked brown rice.

9. Garnish with sesame seeds and chopped green onions before serving.

Cilantro Lime Chicken Fajita Bowl

Preparation Time: 30 minutes

Servings: 4

Ingredients:

- 1.5 lbs boneless, skinless chicken breasts, sliced
- 1 red bell pepper, sliced
- 1 yellow bell pepper, sliced
- 1 onion, sliced
- 2 tablespoons olive oil
- 2 teaspoons ground cumin
- 2 teaspoons chili powder
- Salt and pepper to taste

- Juice of 2 limes
- 1/4 cup fresh cilantro, chopped
- Cooked brown rice for serving
- Avocado slices for garnish
- Greek yogurt or sour cream for topping

Preparation:

1. In a large skillet, heat olive oil over medium-high heat.
2. Add sliced chicken to the skillet and cook until browned and cooked through.
3. Add sliced bell peppers and onion to the skillet. Sauté until the vegetables are tender-crisp.
4. Season with ground cumin, chili powder, salt, and pepper. Stir well.
5. Pour lime juice over the chicken and vegetables. Toss to coat.
6. Stir in chopped cilantro just before serving.
7. Serve the cilantro lime chicken fajita mixture over cooked brown rice.
8. Garnish with avocado slices and a dollop of Greek yogurt or sour cream.

Spaghetti Aglio e Olio with Cherry Tomatoes

Preparation Time: 20 minutes

Servings: 4

Ingredients:

- 400g (14 oz) spaghetti
- 1/3 cup olive oil
- 4 cloves garlic, thinly sliced
- 1/2 teaspoon red pepper flakes (adjust to taste)
- 1 cup cherry tomatoes, halved
- Salt and black pepper to taste
- Fresh parsley, chopped, for garnish
- Grated Parmesan cheese for serving

Preparation:

1. Cook the spaghetti according to package instructions. Reserve some pasta water before draining.
2. In a large skillet, heat olive oil over medium heat.
3. Add thinly sliced garlic and red pepper flakes. Sauté until the garlic is golden but not burnt.
4. Add halved cherry tomatoes to the skillet. Cook for a few minutes until they start to soften.
5. Season with salt and black pepper.
6. Toss the cooked spaghetti into the skillet, coating it with the garlic and oil mixture. Add a bit of pasta water if needed.
7. Garnish with chopped fresh parsley and serve with grated Parmesan cheese.

Baked Cod with Lemon Herb Crust

Preparation Time: 25 minutes

Servings: 2

Ingredients:

- 2 cod fillets
- 1/2 cup breadcrumbs
- 2 tablespoons fresh parsley, chopped
- 1 tablespoon fresh thyme, chopped
- Zest of 1 lemon
- 2 tablespoons melted butter
- Salt and black pepper to taste
- Lemon wedges for serving

Preparation:

1. Preheat the oven to 400°F (200°C).
2. In a bowl, mix breadcrumbs, chopped parsley, chopped thyme, lemon zest, melted butter, salt, and black pepper.
3. Place cod fillets on a baking sheet lined with parchment paper.
4. Press the breadcrumb mixture onto the top of each cod fillet, creating a crust.
5. Bake in the preheated oven for about 15-18 minutes or until the fish is cooked through and the crust is golden brown.
6. Serve the baked cod with lemon wedges.

Butternut Squash and Sage Risotto

Preparation Time: 40 minutes

Servings: 4

Ingredients:

- 1 cup Arborio rice
- 1/2 butternut squash, peeled and diced
- 1 onion, finely chopped
- 3 cloves garlic, minced
- 1/2 cup dry white wine
- 4 cups vegetable broth, kept warm
- 1/2 cup Parmesan cheese, grated
- 2 tablespoons fresh sage, chopped
- 2 tablespoons butter
- Salt and black pepper to taste

Preparation:

1. In a large pan, sauté chopped onion in butter until softened.
2. Add minced garlic and Arborio rice. Cook for 2-3 minutes until the rice is lightly toasted.
3. Pour in the white wine and cook until it's mostly evaporated.
4. Begin adding warm vegetable broth, one ladle at a time, stirring frequently. Allow the liquid to be absorbed before adding more.
5. In the meantime, steam or roast the diced butternut squash until tender.
6. When the risotto is almost cooked (after about 18-20 minutes), stir in the cooked butternut squash, grated Parmesan, and chopped sage.

7. Continue to cook until the rice is creamy and al dente.

8. Season with salt and black pepper to taste.

9. Serve the butternut squash and sage risotto hot.

Mushroom and Spinach Stuffed Chicken Breast

Preparation Time: 35 minutes

Servings: 2

Ingredients:
- 2 boneless, skinless chicken breasts
- 1 cup mushrooms, finely chopped
- 2 cups fresh spinach, chopped
- 2 cloves garlic, minced
- 1/2 cup feta cheese, crumbled
- 1 tablespoon olive oil
- 1 teaspoon dried oregano
- Salt and black pepper to taste
- Toothpicks for securing

Preparation:
1. Preheat the oven to 375°F (190°C).
2. In a skillet, heat olive oil over medium heat. Add minced garlic and sauté until fragrant.
3. Add chopped mushrooms and cook until they release their moisture.

4. Stir in chopped spinach and cook until wilted.

5. Remove the skillet from heat and let the mixture cool slightly.

6. Stir in crumbled feta cheese, dried oregano, salt, and black pepper.

7. Cut a pocket into each chicken breast without cutting all the way through.

8. Stuff each chicken breast with the mushroom and spinach mixture.

9. Secure the openings with toothpicks.

10. Place the stuffed chicken breasts in a baking dish and bake for 25-30 minutes or until the chicken is cooked through.

11. Remove toothpicks before serving.

Black Bean and Sweet Potato Enchiladas

Preparation Time: 45 minutes

Servings: 4

Ingredients:

- 8 small whole wheat or corn tortillas
- 2 cups sweet potatoes, cooked and mashed
- 1 can (15 oz) black beans, drained and rinsed
- 1 cup corn kernels (fresh or frozen)
- 1 cup enchilada sauce
- 1 cup shredded cheese (cheddar or Mexican blend)
- 1 teaspoon ground cumin
- 1 teaspoon chili powder

- 1/2 teaspoon garlic powder
- Salt and black pepper to taste
- Fresh cilantro for garnish
- Greek yogurt or sour cream for topping

Preparation:

1. Preheat the oven to 375°F (190°C).
2. In a bowl, mix mashed sweet potatoes, black beans, corn, ground cumin, chili powder, garlic powder, salt, and black pepper.
3. Warm the tortillas to make them pliable.
4. Spread a portion of the sweet potato mixture onto each tortilla and roll it up.
5. Place the rolled enchiladas in a baking dish.
6. Pour enchilada sauce over the rolled tortillas, ensuring they are well-covered.
7. Sprinkle shredded cheese over the top.
8. Bake in the preheated oven for 20-25 minutes or until the cheese is melted and bubbly.
9. Garnish with fresh cilantro and serve with a dollop of Greek yogurt or sour cream.

Cauliflower Steak with Chimichurri Sauce

Preparation Time: 30 minutes

Servings: 2

Ingredients:

- 1 large cauliflower head
- 2 tablespoons olive oil
- Salt and black pepper to taste

Chimichurri Sauce:

- 1 cup fresh parsley, chopped
- 1/4 cup fresh cilantro, chopped
- 2 cloves garlic, minced
- 1/2 cup olive oil
- 2 tablespoons red wine vinegar
- 1 teaspoon dried oregano
- Salt and black pepper to taste
- Red pepper flakes for a hint of spice (optional)

Preparation:

1. Preheat the oven to 400°F (200°C).
2. Trim the leaves and stem from the cauliflower head, leaving the core intact.
3. Slice the cauliflower into 1-inch thick steaks.
4. Place the cauliflower steaks on a baking sheet.
5. Brush each side of the cauliflower steaks with olive oil and season with salt and black pepper.
6. Roast in the preheated oven for 20-25 minutes or until the cauliflower is tender and golden brown at the edges.

7. While the cauliflower is roasting, prepare the chimichurri sauce by combining chopped parsley, chopped cilantro, minced garlic, olive oil, red wine vinegar, dried oregano, salt, black pepper, and red pepper flakes (if using) in a bowl.

8. Serve the roasted cauliflower steaks drizzled with chimichurri sauce.

Pesto Shrimp and Zucchini Noodles

Preparation Time: 20 minutes

Servings: 2

Ingredients:

- 8 oz shrimp, peeled and deveined
- 2 medium zucchini, spiralized into noodles
- 1/4 cup pesto sauce
- 2 tablespoons olive oil
- 2 cloves garlic, minced
- 1/2 teaspoon red pepper flakes (optional)
- Salt and black pepper to taste
- Cherry tomatoes for garnish
- Fresh basil leaves for garnish
- Grated Parmesan cheese for serving

Preparation:

1. In a large skillet, heat olive oil over medium-high heat.

2. Add minced garlic and red pepper flakes (if using). Sauté until the garlic is fragrant.

3. Add shrimp to the skillet and cook until they turn pink and opaque.

4. Stir in pesto sauce, coating the shrimp evenly.

5. Toss the spiralized zucchini noodles into the skillet. Cook for 2-3 minutes until the noodles are just tender.

6. Season with salt and black pepper to taste.

7. Garnish with cherry tomatoes, fresh basil leaves, and grated Parmesan cheese.

8. Serve the pesto shrimp and zucchini noodles immediately.

Quinoa and Kale Stuffed Acorn Squash

Preparation Time: 45 minutes

Servings: 4

Ingredients:

- 2 acorn squash, halved and seeds removed
- 1 cup quinoa, cooked
- 2 cups kale, chopped
- 1 can (15 oz) chickpeas, drained and rinsed
- 1/2 cup feta cheese, crumbled
- 1/4 cup dried cranberries
- 2 tablespoons olive oil
- 1 tablespoon balsamic vinegar

- 1 teaspoon Dijon mustard
- Salt and black pepper to taste
- Chopped pecans for garnish

Preparation:

1. Preheat the oven to 400°F (200°C).
2. Place acorn squash halves on a baking sheet and cut side down. Roast for 25-30 minutes or until tender.
3. While the squash is roasting, heat olive oil in a skillet over medium heat.
4. Add chopped kale to the skillet and sauté until wilted.
5. In a large bowl, combine cooked quinoa, sautéed kale, chickpeas, feta cheese, and dried cranberries.
6. In a small bowl, whisk together olive oil, balsamic vinegar, Dijon mustard, salt, and black pepper.
7. Pour the dressing over the quinoa mixture and toss to coat.
8. Once the acorn squash halves are tender, stuff them with the quinoa and kale mixture.
9. Garnish with chopped pecans before serving.

Chapter 6: Snack Smart

Hummus and Veggie Sticks

Preparation Time: 15 minutes

Servings: 4

Ingredients:

- 1 can (15 oz) chickpeas, drained and rinsed
- 1/4 cup tahini
- 2 tablespoons lemon juice
- 2 cloves garlic, minced
- 1/2 teaspoon ground cumin
- 1/4 teaspoon paprika
- 1/4 cup extra-virgin olive oil
- Salt and pepper, to taste
- Assorted veggies for dipping (carrot sticks, cucumber slices, bell pepper strips, cherry tomatoes)

Preparation:

1. In a food processor, combine the chickpeas, tahini, lemon juice, garlic, cumin, and paprika.
2. Pulse the ingredients until well combined and slightly smooth.

3. While the food processor is running, slowly drizzle in the olive oil until the hummus reaches a creamy consistency.

4. Season with salt and pepper to taste. Adjust the ingredients as needed, adding more lemon juice or olive oil if desired.

5. Transfer the hummus to a serving bowl and refrigerate for at least 30 minutes before serving.

6. Wash and prepare the assorted veggies for dipping.

7. Serve the hummus with the veggie sticks and enjoy!

Greek Yogurt Parfait with Berries and Granola

Preparation Time: 10 minutes

Servings: 2

Ingredients:

- 1 cup Greek yogurt
- 1 cup mixed berries (strawberries, blueberries, raspberries)
- 1/2 cup granola
- 2 tablespoons honey
- 1/4 cup chopped nuts (optional, for garnish)

Preparation:

1. In two serving glasses or bowls, layer half of the Greek yogurt at the bottom of each.

2. Add a layer of mixed berries on top of the yogurt in each glass.

3. Sprinkle a portion of granola over the berries in each glass.

4. Drizzle 1 tablespoon of honey over each parfait.

5. Repeat the layers, finishing with a final drizzle of honey and a sprinkle of chopped nuts if desired.

6. Serve immediately and enjoy this refreshing Greek Yogurt Parfait with Berries and Granola.

Apple Slices with Almond Butter

Preparation Time: 5 minutes

Servings: 2

Ingredients:

- 2 apples, cored and sliced
- 1/4 cup almond butter
- 1 tablespoon honey
- 1/2 teaspoon cinnamon (optional, for garnish)

Preparation:

1. Arrange the apple slices on a serving plate.

2. In a small microwave-safe bowl, warm the almond butter for 15-20 seconds until it becomes more spreadable.

3. Drizzle the almond butter over the apple slices.

4. Drizzle honey over the almond butter.

5. Optionally, sprinkle cinnamon on top for added flavor.

6. Serve immediately, and enjoy the delightful combination of Apple Slices with Almond Butter.

Trail Mix with Nuts, Seeds, and Dried Fruit

Preparation Time: 5 minutes

Servings: 4

Ingredients:

- 1 cup almonds
- 1 cup walnuts
- 1/2 cup pumpkin seeds
- 1/2 cup sunflower seeds
- 1/2 cup dried cranberries
- 1/2 cup raisins
- 1/2 cup dark chocolate chips

Preparation:

1. In a large mixing bowl, combine almonds, walnuts, pumpkin seeds, sunflower seeds, dried cranberries, raisins, and dark chocolate chips.
2. Toss the ingredients together until well mixed.
3. Divide the trail mix into individual serving portions.
4. Store in an airtight container for a quick and nutritious snack on the go.

Cucumber and Feta Bites

Preparation Time: 10 minutes

Servings: 4

Ingredients:

- 2 cucumbers, sliced into rounds
- 1 cup cherry tomatoes, halved
- 1/2 cup feta cheese, crumbled
- Fresh basil leaves, for garnish
- Balsamic glaze, for drizzling

Preparation:

1. Place cucumber rounds on a serving platter.
2. Top each cucumber round with a cherry tomato half.
3. Sprinkle crumbled feta over the tomatoes.
4. Garnish each bite with a fresh basil leaf.
5. Drizzle balsamic glaze over the cucumber and feta bites.
6. Serve and enjoy these refreshing and savory bites.

Energy-Boosting Smoothie with Spinach and Banana

Preparation Time: 5 minutes

Servings: 2

Ingredients:

- 2 cups fresh spinach leaves
- 1 banana, peeled and sliced
- 1/2 cup Greek yogurt
- 1/2 cup almond milk
- 1 tablespoon chia seeds
- 1 tablespoon honey
- Ice cubes (optional)

Preparation:

1. In a blender, combine fresh spinach, banana slices, Greek yogurt, almond milk, chia seeds, and honey.
2. Blend until smooth and creamy. Add ice cubes if a colder consistency is desired.
3. Pour the smoothie into glasses and serve immediately for a nutritious and energy-boosting drink.

Roasted Chickpeas with Paprika and Garlic

Preparation Time: 40 minutes

Servings: 4

Ingredients:

- 2 cans (15 oz each) chickpeas, drained and rinsed
- 2 tablespoons olive oil
- 1 teaspoon smoked paprika
- 1 teaspoon garlic powder
- Salt and pepper, to taste

Preparation:

1. Preheat the oven to 400°F (200°C).
2. Rinse and drain the chickpeas, then pat them dry with a paper towel.
3. In a bowl, toss chickpeas with olive oil, smoked paprika, garlic powder, salt, and pepper until evenly coated.
4. Spread the seasoned chickpeas on a baking sheet in a single layer.
5. Roast in the preheated oven for 30-35 minutes or until crispy, shaking the pan halfway through for even roasting.
6. Allow the roasted chickpeas to cool before serving.

Whole Grain Crackers with Avocado and Cherry Tomatoes

Preparation Time: 10 minutes

Servings: 4

Ingredients:

- 1 avocado, mashed
- 1 cup cherry tomatoes, halved

- Whole grain crackers

Preparation:

1. Spread a generous amount of mashed avocado on each whole-grain cracker.
2. Top with halved cherry tomatoes.
3. Arrange the crackers on a serving platter and serve immediately.

Cheese and Whole Wheat Pita Wedges

Preparation Time: 15 minutes

Servings: 4

Ingredients:

- 1 cup cheese (cheddar, mozzarella, or your choice), cubed
- 4 whole wheat pita bread rounds, cut into wedges

Preparation:

1. Preheat the oven to 350°F (175°C).
2. Arrange the pita wedges on a baking sheet.
3. Place a cube of cheese on each wedge.
4. Bake in the preheated oven for 10-12 minutes or until the cheese is melted and the edges of the pita are crispy.
5. Serve the cheese and whole wheat pita wedges warm.

Dark Chocolate-Dipped Strawberries

Preparation Time: 20 minutes

Servings: 4

Ingredients:

- 1 cup dark chocolate chips
- 1 pint fresh strawberries, washed and dried

Preparation:

1. In a microwave-safe bowl, melt the dark chocolate chips in 20-second intervals, stirring between each interval until smooth.
2. Hold each strawberry by the stem and dip it into the melted chocolate, coating it halfway.
3. Place the dipped strawberries on a parchment paper-lined tray.
4. Allow the chocolate to set at room temperature or place the tray in the refrigerator for faster setting.
5. Serve the dark chocolate-dipped strawberries once the chocolate is firm. Enjoy!

Chapter 7: Divine Desserts

Classic Chocolate Chip Cookies

Preparation Time: 15 minutes

Baking Time: 10-12 minutes

Servings: 24 cookies

Ingredients:

- 1 cup unsalted butter, softened
- 3/4 cup granulated sugar
- 3/4 cup packed brown sugar
- 2 large eggs
- 1 teaspoon vanilla extract
- 2 1/4 cups all-purpose flour
- 1 teaspoon baking soda
- 1/2 teaspoon salt
- 2 cups chocolate chips

Preparation:

1. Preheat the oven to 375°F (190°C) and line baking sheets with parchment paper.

2. In a large bowl, cream together the softened butter, granulated sugar, and brown sugar until smooth.

3. Beat in the eggs one at a time, then stir in the vanilla extract.

4. In a separate bowl, whisk together the flour, baking soda, and salt. Gradually add this dry mixture to the wet ingredients, mixing until well combined.

5. Fold in the chocolate chips.

6. Drop rounded tablespoons of cookie dough onto the prepared baking sheets.

7. Bake in the preheated oven for 10-12 minutes or until the edges are golden brown.

8. Allow the cookies to cool on the baking sheets for a few minutes before transferring them to a wire rack to cool completely.

Berry-Licious Fruit Salad with Honey-Lime Drizzle

Preparation Time: 15 minutes

Servings: 6

Ingredients:

- 2 cups strawberries, hulled and halved
- 1 cup blueberries
- 1 cup raspberries
- 1 cup blackberries
- 2 tablespoons honey

- Juice of 1 lime
- Fresh mint leaves for garnish

Preparation:

1. In a large bowl, combine strawberries, blueberries, raspberries, and blackberries.
2. In a small bowl, whisk together honey and lime juice.
3. Drizzle the honey-lime mixture over the berries and gently toss to combine.
4. Garnish with fresh mint leaves.
5. Serve immediately or refrigerate until ready to serve.

Decadent Dark Chocolate Avocado Mousse

Preparation Time: 10 minutes

Servings: 4

Ingredients:

- 2 ripe avocados, peeled and pitted
- 1/2 cup cocoa powder
- 1/2 cup maple syrup or agave nectar
- 1 teaspoon vanilla extract
- Pinch of salt
- 1/4 cup almond milk (or any milk of choice)

Preparation:

1. In a food processor, combine avocados, cocoa powder, maple syrup, vanilla extract, and a pinch of salt.

2. Blend until smooth and creamy.

3. Add almond milk gradually until the mousse reaches your desired consistency.

4. Spoon the chocolate avocado mousse into serving glasses.

5. Refrigerate for at least 30 minutes before serving.

Baked Apple Crisp with Cinnamon-Oat Topping

Preparation Time: 20 minutes

Baking Time: 40 minutes

Servings: 6

Ingredients:

- 6 apples, peeled, cored, and sliced
- 1 tablespoon lemon juice
- 1/4 cup granulated sugar
- 1 teaspoon ground cinnamon
- 1/2 cup old-fashioned oats
- 1/4 cup all-purpose flour
- 1/4 cup brown sugar
- 1/4 cup unsalted butter, cold and cubed

Preparation:

1. Preheat the oven to 350°F (175°C) and grease a baking dish.

2. In a large bowl, toss apple slices with lemon juice, granulated sugar, and ground cinnamon. Transfer to the prepared baking dish.

3. In a separate bowl, combine oats, flour, brown sugar, and cubed butter. Use your fingers to mix until crumbly.

4. Sprinkle the oat mixture evenly over the apples.

5. Bake in the preheated oven for 40 minutes or until the topping is golden brown and the apples are tender.

6. Allow the baked apple crisp to cool slightly before serving. Enjoy!

Vanilla Bean Panna Cotta with Raspberry Coulis

Preparation Time: 15 minutes

Chilling Time: 4 hours

Servings: 4

Ingredients:

- 2 cups heavy cream
- 1/2 cup granulated sugar
- 1 vanilla bean, split and seeds scraped (or 1 teaspoon vanilla extract)
- 2 1/2 teaspoons gelatin powder
- 3 tablespoons cold water

Raspberry Coulis:

- 1 cup fresh raspberries
- 2 tablespoons powdered sugar
- 1 tablespoon lemon juice

Preparation:

1. In a saucepan, heat the heavy cream, sugar, and vanilla bean seeds (or vanilla extract) over medium heat until it almost comes to a simmer. Remove from heat.
2. In a small bowl, sprinkle gelatin over cold water and let it sit for a few minutes to bloom.
3. Add the bloomed gelatin to the warm cream mixture and stir until completely dissolved.
4. Strain the mixture through a fine-mesh sieve to remove vanilla bean remnants.
5. Pour the mixture into serving glasses or ramekins.
6. Refrigerate for at least 4 hours or until set.

Raspberry Coulis:

- In a blender, combine raspberries, powdered sugar, and lemon juice.
- Blend until smooth.
- Strain the mixture to remove the seeds.
- Refrigerate until ready to serve.
- Drizzle the raspberry coulis over the chilled panna cotta before serving.

Homemade Banana Bread with Walnuts

Preparation Time: 15 minutes

Baking Time: 60 minutes

Servings: 8

Ingredients:

- 3 ripe bananas, mashed
- 1/2 cup unsalted butter, melted
- 1 teaspoon vanilla extract
- 1 teaspoon baking soda
- Pinch of salt
- 3/4 cup granulated sugar
- 1 large egg, beaten
- 1 1/2 cups all-purpose flour
- 1/2 cup chopped walnuts

Preparation:

1. Preheat the oven to 350°F (175°C) and grease a loaf pan.
2. In a mixing bowl, mash the ripe bananas.
3. Stir melted butter into the mashed bananas.
4. Add vanilla extract, baking soda, salt, and sugar. Mix well.
5. Add the beaten egg and mix thoroughly.

6. Stir in the flour until just incorporated, then fold in the chopped walnuts.

7. Pour the batter into the prepared loaf pan.

8. Bake in the preheated oven for about 60 minutes or until a toothpick inserted into the center comes out clean.

9. Allow the banana bread to cool before slicing.

Strawberry Shortcake Parfait

Preparation Time: 15 minutes

Servings: 4

Ingredients:

- 2 cups fresh strawberries, hulled and sliced
- 1/4 cup granulated sugar
- 1 cup whipped cream or vanilla yogurt
- 2 cups shortcake or pound cake, cubed

Preparation:

1. In a bowl, toss sliced strawberries with granulated sugar. Let them sit for a few minutes until the juices are released.

2. In serving glasses, layer cubed shortcake or pound cake, followed by a spoonful of strawberries and a dollop of whipped cream or vanilla yogurt.

3. Repeat the layers until the glasses are filled.

4. Garnish with a strawberry on top.

5. Serve immediately and enjoy this delightful Strawberry Shortcake Parfait.

Lemon Blueberry Cheesecake Bars

Preparation Time: 20 minutes

Baking Time: 40 minutes

Chilling Time: 4 hours

Servings: 16 bars

Ingredients:

- 1 1/2 cups graham cracker crumbs
- 1/2 cup unsalted butter, melted
- 3 packages (8 oz each) of cream cheese, softened
- 1 cup granulated sugar
- 3 large eggs
- 1/4 cup all-purpose flour
- 1 tablespoon lemon zest
- 1/4 cup fresh lemon juice
- 1 cup fresh blueberries

Preparation:

1. Preheat the oven to 325°F (163°C) and line a baking pan with parchment paper.

2. In a bowl, combine graham cracker crumbs and melted butter. Press the mixture into the bottom of the prepared pan to form the crust.

3. In a large mixing bowl, beat cream cheese and sugar until smooth.

4. Add eggs one at a time, beating well after each addition.

5. Mix in flour, lemon zest, and lemon juice until just combined.

6. Gently fold in blueberries.

7. Pour the cream cheese mixture over the crust and spread it evenly.

8. Bake in the preheated oven for 40 minutes or until the center is set.

9. Allow the cheesecake bars to cool completely, then refrigerate for at least 4 hours before cutting into squares.

Pistachio and Raspberry Chocolate Bark

Preparation Time: 15 minutes

Chilling Time: 1 hour

Servings: Varies

Ingredients:

- 12 oz dark chocolate, chopped

- 1/2 cup shelled pistachios, chopped

- 1/2 cup fresh raspberries

Preparation:

1. Line a baking sheet with parchment paper.
2. In a heatproof bowl, melt the dark chocolate using a double boiler or in short bursts in the microwave.
3. Once melted, spread the chocolate onto the prepared baking sheet.
4. Sprinkle chopped pistachios and place raspberries evenly over the melted chocolate.
5. Gently press the toppings into the chocolate.
6. Refrigerate for at least 1 hour or until the chocolate is firm.
7. Break the chocolate bark into pieces and serve. Enjoy the delicious combination of Pistachio and Raspberry Chocolate Bark.

Coconut Chia Seed Pudding with Mango Puree

Preparation Time: 10 minutes

Chilling Time: 4 hours or overnight

Servings: 4

Ingredients:

- 1/2 cup chia seeds
- 2 cups coconut milk (canned or homemade)
- 2 tablespoons maple syrup or honey
- 1 teaspoon vanilla extract
- Pinch of salt

- 1 large ripe mango, peeled and diced

Preparation:

1. In a bowl, combine chia seeds, coconut milk, maple syrup or honey, vanilla extract, and a pinch of salt.

2. Whisk the ingredients together thoroughly, making sure the chia seeds are well distributed.

3. Cover the bowl and refrigerate the mixture for at least 4 hours or overnight to allow the chia seeds to absorb the liquid and create a pudding-like consistency.

4. Before serving, prepare the mango puree by placing the diced mango in a blender or food processor. Blend until smooth.

5. Once the chia pudding has set, stir it well to ensure an even texture.

6. Spoon the coconut chia seed pudding into serving glasses or bowls.

7. Top each serving with a generous spoonful of mango puree.

8. Optionally, garnish with additional diced mango or shredded coconut.

9. Serve chilled and enjoy this delicious and nutritious Coconut Chia Seed Pudding with Mango Puree.

Chapter 8: Refreshing Beverages

Iced Green Tea with Mint and Lemon

Preparation Time: 15 minutes

Chilling Time: 2 hours

Servings: 4

Ingredients:

- 4 green tea bags
- 4 cups water
- 1/4 cup fresh mint leaves
- 1 lemon, sliced
- Ice cubes
- Honey or agave syrup (optional, for sweetness)

Preparation:

1. Bring 4 cups of water to a boil and steep the green tea bags for 3-5 minutes.
2. Remove the tea bags and allow the tea to cool to room temperature.
3. Refrigerate the tea for at least 2 hours to chill.
4. In a pitcher, combine the chilled green tea, fresh mint leaves, and lemon slices.

5. Add ice cubes to the pitcher.

6. If desired, add honey or agave syrup to sweeten the iced tea.

7. Stir well, serve over ice, and enjoy the refreshing Iced Green Tea with Mint and Lemon.

Fresh Watermelon Mint Cooler

Preparation Time: 10 minutes

Chilling Time: 1 hour

Servings: 4

Ingredients:

- 4 cups fresh watermelon, cubed
- 1/4 cup fresh mint leaves
- 1 tablespoon lime juice
- 2 cups cold water
- Ice cubes

Preparation:

1. In a blender, combine fresh watermelon cubes, mint leaves, and lime juice.

2. Blend until smooth.

3. Strain the watermelon mixture into a pitcher to remove pulp, if desired.

4. Add cold water to the pitcher and stir well.

5. Refrigerate for at least 1 hour to chill.

6. Serve over ice and garnish with mint leaves.

7. Enjoy the cooling and hydrating Fresh Watermelon Mint Cooler.

Homemade Ginger Lemonade

Preparation Time: 15 minutes

Chilling Time: 1 hour

Servings: 6

Ingredients:

- 1 cup fresh lemon juice (about 6 lemons)
- 1/2 cup granulated sugar
- 1 tablespoon fresh ginger, grated
- 6 cups cold water
- Ice cubes
- Lemon slices and fresh mint for garnish

Preparation:

1. In a small saucepan, combine sugar and 1 cup of water. Heat over medium heat until the sugar dissolves, stirring occasionally.

2. Add grated ginger to the sugar-water mixture and let it simmer for 5 minutes. Remove from heat and let it cool.

3. In a large pitcher, combine fresh lemon juice and the ginger-infused sugar water.

4. Add 6 cups of cold water and stir well.

5. Refrigerate for at least 1 hour to chill.

6. Serve the Ginger Lemonade over ice and garnish with lemon slices and fresh mint.

7. Enjoy the zesty and invigorating Homemade Ginger Lemonade.

Cucumber Basil Sparkling Water

Preparation Time: 10 minutes

Servings: 4

Ingredients:
- 1 cucumber, thinly sliced
- Handful of fresh basil leaves
- 4 cups sparkling water
- Ice cubes
- Lemon slices (optional, for garnish)

Preparation:
1. In a pitcher, combine cucumber slices and fresh basil leaves.
2. Pour sparkling water over the cucumber and basil mixture.
3. Stir gently and refrigerate for 10 minutes to infuse flavors.
4. Fill glasses with ice cubes.

5. Pour the cucumber basil-infused sparkling water over the ice.

6. Garnish with lemon slices if desired.

7. Serve immediately and enjoy the crisp and refreshing Cucumber Basil Sparkling Water.

Golden Turmeric Latte

Preparation Time: 10 minutes

Servings: 2

Ingredients:

- 2 cups milk (dairy or plant-based)
- 1 teaspoon ground turmeric
- 1/2 teaspoon ground cinnamon
- 1/4 teaspoon ground ginger
- 1 tablespoon honey or maple syrup
- 1 teaspoon coconut oil (optional)
- Pinch of black pepper (enhances turmeric absorption)

Preparation:

1. In a small saucepan, heat the milk over medium heat until it's warm but not boiling.

2. Whisk in the ground turmeric, cinnamon, ground ginger, honey or maple syrup, and coconut oil (if using).

3. Continue to whisk until the mixture is well combined and heated through.

4. Add a pinch of black pepper and stir.

5. Pour the golden turmeric latte into mugs and enjoy the warm and comforting beverage.

Raspberry Hibiscus Iced Tea

Preparation Time: 15 minutes

Chilling Time: 2 hours

Servings: 4

Ingredients:

- 4 hibiscus tea bags
- 4 cups boiling water
- 1/4 cup honey or agave syrup
- 1 cup fresh raspberries
- Ice cubes
- Lemon slices (optional, for garnish)

Preparation:

1. Place hibiscus tea bags in a heatproof pitcher.

2. Pour boiling water over the tea bags and let it steep for about 10 minutes.

3. Remove the tea bags and stir in honey or agave syrup.

4. Allow the tea to cool to room temperature, then refrigerate for at least 2 hours.

5. Before serving, add fresh raspberries to the tea.

6. Serve over ice and garnish with lemon slices if desired.

7. Enjoy the refreshing Raspberry Hibiscus Iced Tea.

Mango Coconut Smoothie

Preparation Time: 5 minutes

Servings: 2

Ingredients:

- 1 cup frozen mango chunks
- 1/2 cup coconut milk
- 1/2 cup Greek yogurt
- 1 tablespoon honey or agave syrup
- Ice cubes (optional)

Preparation:

1. In a blender, combine frozen mango chunks, coconut milk, Greek yogurt, and honey or agave syrup.

2. Blend until smooth and creamy.

3. If a thicker consistency is desired, add ice cubes and blend again.

4. Pour the mango coconut smoothie into glasses and enjoy this tropical and satisfying beverage.

Sparkling Lavender Lemonade

Preparation Time: 15 minutes

Chilling Time: 1 hour

Servings: 4

Ingredients:

- 1 cup fresh lemon juice (about 6 lemons)
- 1/2 cup granulated sugar
- 1 tablespoon dried lavender buds
- 4 cups cold sparkling water
- Ice cubes
- Lemon slices and fresh lavender sprigs for garnish

Preparation:

1. In a small saucepan, combine sugar and 1 cup of water. Heat over medium heat until the sugar dissolves, stirring occasionally.
2. Remove from heat and add dried lavender buds. Let it steep for 10 minutes, then strain to remove the lavender.
3. In a pitcher, combine fresh lemon juice, lavender-infused sugar water, and cold sparkling water.

4. Stir well and refrigerate for at least 1 hour to chill.

5. Serve the sparkling lavender lemonade over ice, garnished with lemon slices and fresh lavender sprigs.

6. Enjoy the floral and effervescent Sparkling Lavender Lemonade.

Cold Brew Coffee with Vanilla Almond Milk

Preparation Time: 5 minutes

Chilling Time: 12-24 hours

Servings: 2

Ingredients:

- 1/2 cup coarsely ground coffee
- 2 cups cold water
- 1 cup vanilla almond milk
- Ice cubes
- Sweetener of choice (optional)

Preparation:

1. In a jar or French press, combine coarsely ground coffee and cold water.

2. Stir to ensure all coffee grounds are saturated, then cover and refrigerate for 12-24 hours.

3. After steeping, strain the cold brew concentrate through a fine-mesh sieve or coffee filter.

4. To serve, fill glasses with ice cubes and pour the cold brew concentrate over the ice.

5. Add vanilla almond milk to each glass, adjusting the ratio to your preference.

6. If desired, sweeten the cold brew with your choice of sweetener.

7. Stir well and enjoy the smooth and creamy Cold Brew Coffee with Vanilla Almond Milk.

Pineapple Ginger Kombucha

Preparation Time: 10 minutes

Fermentation Time: 7-14 days

Servings: Varies

Ingredients:
- 4 cups brewed green or black tea
- 1 cup granulated sugar
- 1 SCOBY (Symbiotic Culture Of Bacteria and Yeast)
- 1 cup plain, unflavored kombucha (as a starter)
- 1 cup pineapple juice
- 1 tablespoon freshly grated ginger

Preparation:

1. Brew tea and dissolve sugar in it. Let it cool to room temperature.
2. In a clean glass container, combine the cooled tea, SCOBY, plain kombucha, pineapple juice, and grated ginger.
3. Cover the container with a breathable cloth or coffee filter and secure it with a rubber band.
4. Place the container in a warm, dark place for 7-14 days to ferment. Taste the kombucha periodically to check its flavor.
5. Once the kombucha reaches the desired level of fermentation, remove the SCOBY.
6. Strain the kombucha to remove ginger and any sediment.
7. Bottle the kombucha and refrigerate to chill.
8. Serve the Pineapple Ginger Kombucha over ice and enjoy the fizzy and flavorful beverage.

Chapter 9: Weekly Meal Plan

Embark on a journey of organized and health-conscious eating with this weekly meal plan. Designed to provide a balanced and delicious approach to nourishing your body, the following plan offers a variety of recipes to suit different tastes and dietary preferences. Use this guide to simplify your weekly meal preparation and enjoy the benefits of thoughtful and nutritious eating.

30-Day Meal Plan

Day 1:

Breakfast: Berry Power Smoothie Bowl

Calories: 350 | Protein: 15g | Carbs: 45g | Fat: 12g

Lunch: Mediterranean Quinoa Salad

Calories: 420 | Protein: 18g | Carbs: 55g | Fat: 16g

Dinner: Lemon Garlic Roasted Chicken with Rosemary Potatoes

Calories: 480 | Protein: 30g | Carbs: 35g | Fat: 22g

Snack: Hummus and Veggie Sticks

Calories: 150 | Protein: 5g | Carbs: 20g | Fat: 7g

Dessert: Classic Chocolate Chip Cookies

Calories: 120 | Protein: 2g | Carbs: 15g | Fat: 6g

Beverage: Iced Green Tea with Mint and Lemon

Calories: 0 | Protein: 0g | Carbs: 0g | Fat: 0g

Day 2:

Breakfast: Avocado Toast with Poached Egg

Calories: 320 | Protein: 12g | Carbs: 30g | Fat: 18g

Lunch: Grilled Chicken and Avocado Wrap

Calories: 380 | Protein: 25g | Carbs: 30g | Fat: 16g

Dinner: Shrimp and Quinoa Stuffed Bell Peppers

Calories: 430 | Protein: 20g | Carbs: 40g | Fat: 20g

Snack: Greek Yogurt Parfait with Berries and Granola

Calories: 280 | Protein: 15g | Carbs: 25g | Fat: 14g

Dessert: Berry-Licious Fruit Salad with Honey-Lime Drizzle

Calories: 90 | Protein: 1g | Carbs: 22g | Fat: 0g

Beverage: Fresh Watermelon Mint Cooler

Calories: 30 | Protein: 0g | Carbs: 8g | Fat: 0g

Day 3:

Breakfast: Quinoa Breakfast Bowl

Calories: 300 | Protein: 10g | Carbs: 40g | Fat: 12g

Lunch: Vegetarian Buddha Bowl with Tahini Dressing

Calories: 420 | Protein: 15g | Carbs: 50g | Fat: 18g

Dinner: Vegetarian Chickpea Tikka Masala

Calories: 380 | Protein: 18g | Carbs: 35g | Fat: 15g

Snack: Apple Slices with Almond Butter

Calories: 200 | Protein: 5g | Carbs: 25g | Fat: 10g

Dessert: Decadent Dark Chocolate Avocado Mousse

Calories: 150 | Protein: 3g | Carbs: 12g | Fat: 10g

Beverage: Homemade Ginger Lemonade

Calories: 50 | Protein: 0g | Carbs: 15g | Fat: 0g

Day 4:

Breakfast: Greek Yogurt Parfait

Calories: 280 | Protein: 15g | Carbs: 30g | Fat: 12g

Lunch: Salmon and Asparagus Foil Pack

Calories: 450 | Protein: 30g | Carbs: 25g | Fat: 22g

Dinner: Grilled Salmon with Dill Yogurt Sauce

Calories: 380 | Protein: 25g | Carbs: 20g | Fat: 18g

Snack: Trail Mix with Nuts, Seeds, and Dried Fruit

Calories: 220 | Protein: 10g | Carbs: 15g | Fat: 14g

Dessert: Baked Apple Crisp with Cinnamon-Oat Topping

Calories: 180 | Protein: 2g | Carbs: 40g | Fat: 4g

Beverage: Cucumber Basil Sparkling Water

Calories: 0 | Protein: 0g | Carbs: 0g | Fat: 0g

Day 5:

Breakfast: Spinach and Feta Omelette

Calories: 320 | Protein: 20g | Carbs: 15g | Fat: 22g

Lunch: Caprese Stuffed Portobello Mushrooms

Calories: 350 | Protein: 12g | Carbs: 25g | Fat: 18g

Dinner: Eggplant Parmesan with Whole Wheat Pasta

Calories: 430 | Protein: 20g | Carbs: 40g | Fat: 20g

Snack: Cucumber and Feta Bites

Calories: 150 | Protein: 8g | Carbs: 10g | Fat: 10g

Dessert: Vanilla Bean Panna Cotta with Raspberry Coulis

Calories: 200 | Protein: 3g | Carbs: 30g | Fat: 8g

Beverage: Golden Turmeric Latte

Calories: 40 | Protein: 1g | Carbs: 8g | Fat: 0g

Day 6:

Breakfast: Chia Seed Pudding

Calories: 250 | Protein: 8g | Carbs: 30g | Fat: 12g

Lunch: Teriyaki Tofu Stir-Fry with Broccoli and Bell Peppers

Calories: 400 | Protein: 15g | Carbs: 35g | Fat: 18g

Dinner: Cilantro Lime Chicken Fajita Bowl

Calories: 380 | Protein: 25g | Carbs: 30g | Fat: 15g

Snack: Energy-boosting smoothie with Spinach and Banana

Calories: 230 | Protein: 12g | Carbs: 30g | Fat: 8g

Dessert: Pistachio and Raspberry Chocolate Bark

Calories: 150 | Protein: 3g | Carbs: 15g | Fat: 10g

Beverage: Raspberry Hibiscus Iced Tea

Calories: 20 | Protein: 0g | Carbs: 5g | Fat: 0g

Day 7:

Breakfast: Banana Nut Oatmeal

Calories: 290 | Protein: 10g | Carbs: 45g | Fat: 8g

Lunch: Sweet Potato and Black Bean Quesadillas

Calories: 370 | Protein: 15g | Carbs: 40g | Fat: 18g

Dinner: Butternut Squash and Sage Risotto

Calories: 410 | Protein: 10g | Carbs: 60g | Fat: 15g

Snack: Dark Chocolate-Dipped Strawberries

Calories: 120 | Protein: 1g | Carbs: 25g | Fat: 5g

Dessert: Coconut Chia Seed Pudding with Mango Puree

Calories: 180 | Protein: 4g | Carbs: 25g | Fat: 8g

Beverage: Mango Coconut Smoothie

Calories: 150 | Protein: 2g | Carbs: 30g | Fat: 5g

Day 8:

Breakfast: Cottage Cheese and Pineapple Bowl

Calories: 280 | Protein: 15g | Carbs: 30g | Fat: 12g

Lunch: Cauliflower Fried Rice with Shrimp

Calories: 420 | Protein: 30g | Carbs: 35g | Fat: 16g

Dinner: Mushroom and Spinach Stuffed Chicken Breast

Calories: 380 | Protein: 35g | Carbs: 15g | Fat: 18g

Snack: Roasted Chickpeas with Paprika and Garlic

Calories: 160 | Protein: 6g | Carbs: 22g | Fat: 6g

Dessert: Classic Chocolate Chip Cookies

Calories: 120 | Protein: 2g | Carbs: 15g | Fat: 6g

Beverage: Sparkling Lavender Lemonade

Calories: 40 | Protein: 0g | Carbs: 10g | Fat: 0g

Day 9:

Breakfast: Sweet Potato Breakfast Hash

Calories: 300 | Protein: 8g | Carbs: 45g | Fat: 12g

Lunch: Mango Avocado Chicken Salad

Calories: 360 | Protein: 25g | Carbs: 30g | Fat: 16g

Dinner: Black Bean and Sweet Potato Enchiladas

Calories: 430 | Protein: 15g | Carbs: 50g | Fat: 20g

Snack: Whole Grain Crackers with Avocado and Cherry Tomatoes

Calories: 200 | Protein: 5g | Carbs: 20g | Fat: 12g

Dessert: Berry-Licious Fruit Salad with Honey-Lime Drizzle

Calories: 90 | Protein: 1g | Carbs: 22g | Fat: 0g

Beverage: Cold Brew Coffee with Vanilla Almond Milk

Calories: 30 | Protein: 1g | Carbs: 4g | Fat: 1g

Day 10:

Breakfast: Blueberry Almond Overnight Oats

Calories: 280 | Protein: 10g | Carbs: 40g | Fat: 10g

Lunch: Tomato Basil Mozzarella Panini

Calories: 340 | Protein: 15g | Carbs: 35g | Fat: 16g

Dinner: Cauliflower Steak with Chimichurri Sauce

Calories: 370 | Protein: 15g | Carbs: 40g | Fat: 18g

Snack: Cheese and Whole Wheat Pita Wedges

Calories: 220 | Protein: 10g | Carbs: 15g | Fat: 14g

Dessert: Decadent Dark Chocolate Avocado Mousse

Calories: 150 | Protein: 3g | Carbs: 12g | Fat: 10g

Beverage: Pineapple Ginger Kombucha

Calories: 40 | Protein: 0g | Carbs: 10g | Fat: 0g

Day 11:

Breakfast: Egg White Veggie Scramble

Calories: 250 | Protein: 15g | Carbs: 10g | Fat: 18g

Lunch: Lentil and Vegetable Soup

Calories: 320 | Protein: 15g | Carbs: 55g | Fat: 6g

Dinner: Pesto Zucchini Noodles with Cherry Tomatoes

Calories: 380 | Protein: 10g | Carbs: 30g | Fat: 22g

Snack: Energy-boosting smoothie with Spinach and Banana

Calories: 230 | Protein: 12g | Carbs: 30g | Fat: 8g

Dessert: Baked Apple Crisp with Cinnamon-Oat Topping

Calories: 180 | Protein: 2g | Carbs: 40g | Fat: 4g

Beverage: Raspberry Hibiscus Iced Tea

Calories: 20 | Protein: 0g | Carbs: 5g | Fat: 0g

Day 12:

Breakfast: Apple Cinnamon Quinoa Porridge

Calories: 300 | Protein: 8g | Carbs: 55g | Fat: 6g

Lunch: Quinoa and Roasted Vegetable Stuffed Peppers

Calories: 420 | Protein: 15g | Carbs: 60g | Fat: 18g

Dinner: Lemon Garlic Roasted Chicken with Rosemary Potatoes

Calories: 480 | Protein: 30g | Carbs: 35g | Fat: 22g

Snack: Trail Mix with Nuts, Seeds, and Dried Fruit

Calories: 220 | Protein: 10g | Carbs: 15g | Fat: 14g

Dessert: Pistachio and Raspberry Chocolate Bark

Calories: 150 | Protein: 3g | Carbs: 15g | Fat: 10g

Beverage: Mango Coconut Smoothie

Calories: 150 | Protein: 2g | Carbs: 30g | Fat: 5g

Day 13:

Breakfast: Smoked Salmon and Cream Cheese Bagel

Calories: 350 | Protein: 20g | Carbs: 30g | Fat: 18g

Lunch: Asian Sesame Ginger Tofu Bowl

Calories: 400 | Protein: 15g | Carbs: 35g | Fat: 20g

Dinner: Shrimp and Quinoa Stuffed Bell Peppers

Calories: 430 | Protein: 20g | Carbs: 40g | Fat: 20g

Snack: Cucumber and Feta Bites

Calories: 150 | Protein: 8g | Carbs: 10g | Fat: 10g

Dessert: Coconut Chia Seed Pudding with Mango Puree

Calories: 180 | Protein: 4g | Carbs: 25g | Fat: 8g

Beverage: Sparkling Lavender Lemonade

Calories: 40 | Protein: 0g | Carbs: 10g | Fat: 0g

Day 14:

Breakfast: Mango Coconut Chia Smoothie

Calories: 280 | Protein: 8g | Carbs: 40g | Fat: 10g

Lunch: Pesto Zucchini Noodles with Cherry Tomatoes

Calories: 340 | Protein: 10g | Carbs: 30g | Fat: 22g

Dinner: Grilled Chicken and Avocado Wrap

Calories: 380 | Protein: 25g | Carbs: 30g | Fat: 16g

Snack: Whole Grain Crackers with Avocado and Cherry Tomatoes

Calories: 220 | Protein: 10g | Carbs: 15g | Fat: 14g

Dessert: Vanilla Bean Panna Cotta with Raspberry Coulis

Calories: 200 | Protein: 3g | Carbs: 30g | Fat: 8g

Beverage: Cold Brew Coffee with Vanilla Almond Milk

Calories: 30 | Protein: 1g | Carbs: 4g | Fat: 1g

Day 15:

Breakfast: Peanut Butter Banana Protein Pancakes

Calories: 320 | Protein: 15g | Carbs: 30g | Fat: 18g

Lunch: Quinoa and Roasted Vegetable Stuffed Peppers

Calories: 420 | Protein: 15g | Carbs: 60g | Fat: 18g

Dinner: Lemon Garlic Roasted Chicken with Rosemary Potatoes

Calories: 480 | Protein: 30g | Carbs: 35g | Fat: 22g

Snack: Hummus and Veggie Sticks

Calories: 150 | Protein: 5g | Carbs: 20g | Fat: 7g

Dessert: Pistachio and Raspberry Chocolate Bark

Calories: 150 | Protein: 3g | Carbs: 15g | Fat: 10g

Beverage: Pineapple Ginger Kombucha

Calories: 40 | Protein: 0g | Carbs: 10g | Fat: 0g

Day 16:

Breakfast: Berry-Licious Fruit Salad with Honey-Lime Drizzle

Calories: 90 | Protein: 1g | Carbs: 22g | Fat: 0g

Lunch: Caprese Stuffed Portobello Mushrooms

Calories: 350 | Protein: 12g | Carbs: 25g | Fat: 18g

Dinner: Butternut Squash and Sage Risotto

Calories: 410 | Protein: 10g | Carbs: 60g | Fat: 15g

Snack: Dark Chocolate-Dipped Strawberries

Calories: 120 | Protein: 1g | Carbs: 25g | Fat: 5g

Dessert: Coconut Chia Seed Pudding with Mango Puree

Calories: 180 | Protein: 4g | Carbs: 25g | Fat: 8g

Beverage: Sparkling Lavender Lemonade

Calories: 40 | Protein: 0g | Carbs: 10g | Fat: 0g

Day 17:

Breakfast: Blueberry Almond Overnight Oats

Calories: 280 | Protein: 10g | Carbs: 40g | Fat: 10g

Lunch: Tomato Basil Mozzarella Panini

Calories: 340 | Protein: 15g | Carbs: 35g | Fat: 16g

Dinner: Cauliflower Steak with Chimichurri Sauce

Calories: 370 | Protein: 15g | Carbs: 40g | Fat: 18g

Snack: Cheese and Whole Wheat Pita Wedges

Calories: 220 | Protein: 10g | Carbs: 15g | Fat: 14g

Dessert: Decadent Dark Chocolate Avocado Mousse

Calories: 150 | Protein: 3g | Carbs: 12g | Fat: 10g

Beverage: Pineapple Ginger Kombucha

Calories: 40 | Protein: 0g | Carbs: 10g | Fat: 0g

Day 18:

Breakfast: Spinach and Feta Omelette

Calories: 320 | Protein: 20g | Carbs: 15g | Fat: 22g

Lunch: Sweet Potato and Black Bean Quesadillas

Calories: 370 | Protein: 15g | Carbs: 40g | Fat: 18g

Dinner: Mushroom and Spinach Stuffed Chicken Breast

Calories: 380 | Protein: 35g | Carbs: 15g | Fat: 18g

Snack: Roasted Chickpeas with Paprika and Garlic

Calories: 160 | Protein: 6g | Carbs: 22g | Fat: 6g

Dessert: Classic Chocolate Chip Cookies

Calories: 120 | Protein: 2g | Carbs: 15g | Fat: 6g

Beverage: Sparkling Lavender Lemonade

Calories: 40 | Protein: 0g | Carbs: 10g | Fat: 0g

Day 19:

Breakfast: Chia Seed Pudding

Calories: 250 | Protein: 8g | Carbs: 30g | Fat: 12g

Lunch: Teriyaki Tofu Stir-Fry with Broccoli and Bell Peppers

Calories: 400 | Protein: 15g | Carbs: 35g | Fat: 18g

Dinner: Cilantro Lime Chicken Fajita Bowl

Calories: 380 | Protein: 25g | Carbs: 30g | Fat: 15g

Snack: Energy-boosting smoothie with Spinach and Banana

Calories: 230 | Protein: 12g | Carbs: 30g | Fat: 8g

Dessert: Pistachio and Raspberry Chocolate Bark

Calories: 150 | Protein: 3g | Carbs: 15g | Fat: 10g

Beverage: Raspberry Hibiscus Iced Tea

Calories: 20 | Protein: 0g | Carbs: 5g | Fat: 0g

Day 20:

Breakfast: Banana Nut Oatmeal

Calories: 290 | Protein: 10g | Carbs: 45g | Fat: 8g

Lunch: Mango Avocado Chicken Salad

Calories: 360 | Protein: 25g | Carbs: 30g | Fat: 16g

Dinner: Black Bean and Sweet Potato Enchiladas

Calories: 430 | Protein: 15g | Carbs: 50g | Fat: 20g

Snack: Whole Grain Crackers with Avocado and Cherry Tomatoes

Calories: 200 | Protein: 5g | Carbs: 20g | Fat: 12g

Dessert: Berry-Licious Fruit Salad with Honey-Lime Drizzle

Calories: 90 | Protein: 1g | Carbs: 22g | Fat: 0g

Beverage: Cold Brew Coffee with Vanilla Almond Milk

Calories: 30 | Protein: 1g | Carbs: 4g | Fat: 1g

Day 21:

Breakfast: Quinoa Breakfast Bowl

Calories: 300 | Protein: 10g | Carbs: 40g | Fat: 12g

Lunch: Vegetarian Buddha Bowl with Tahini Dressing

Calories: 420 | Protein: 15g | Carbs: 50g | Fat: 18g

Dinner: Vegetarian Chickpea Tikka Masala

Calories: 380 | Protein: 18g | Carbs: 35g | Fat: 15g

Snack: Apple Slices with Almond Butter

Calories: 200 | Protein: 5g | Carbs: 25g | Fat: 10g

Dessert: Decadent Dark Chocolate Avocado Mousse

Calories: 150 | Protein: 3g | Carbs: 12g | Fat: 10g

Beverage: Homemade Ginger Lemonade

Calories: 50 | Protein: 0g | Carbs: 15g | Fat: 0g

Day 22:

Breakfast: Greek Yogurt Parfait

Calories: 280 | Protein: 15g | Carbs: 30g | Fat: 12g

Lunch: Cauliflower Fried Rice with Shrimp

Calories: 420 | Protein: 30g | Carbs: 35g | Fat: 16g

Dinner: Mushroom and Spinach Stuffed Chicken Breast

Calories: 380 | Protein: 35g | Carbs: 15g | Fat: 18g

Snack: Roasted Chickpeas with Paprika and Garlic

Calories: 160 | Protein: 6g | Carbs: 22g | Fat: 6g

Dessert: Strawberry Shortcake Parfait

Calories: 200 | Protein: 5g | Carbs: 30g | Fat: 8g

Beverage: Fresh Watermelon Mint Cooler

Calories: 50 | Protein: 1g | Carbs: 12g | Fat: 0g

Day 23:

Breakfast: Smoked Salmon and Cream Cheese Bagel

Calories: 350 | Protein: 20g | Carbs: 30g | Fat: 18g

Lunch: Asian Sesame Ginger Tofu Bowl

Calories: 400 | Protein: 15g | Carbs: 35g | Fat: 20g

Dinner: Shrimp and Quinoa Stuffed Bell Peppers

Calories: 430 | Protein: 20g | Carbs: 40g | Fat: 20g

Snack: Cucumber and Feta Bites

Calories: 150 | Protein: 8g | Carbs: 10g | Fat: 10g

Dessert: Coconut Chia Seed Pudding with Mango Puree

Calories: 180 | Protein: 4g | Carbs: 25g | Fat: 8g

Beverage: Sparkling Lavender Lemonade

Calories: 40 | Protein: 0g | Carbs: 10g | Fat: 0g

Day 24:

Breakfast: Mango Coconut Chia Smoothie

Calories: 280 | Protein: 8g | Carbs: 40g | Fat: 10g

Lunch: Pesto Zucchini Noodles with Cherry Tomatoes

Calories: 340 | Protein: 10g | Carbs: 30g | Fat: 22g

Dinner: Grilled Chicken and Avocado Wrap

Calories: 380 | Protein: 25g | Carbs: 30g | Fat: 16g

Snack: Whole Grain Crackers with Avocado and Cherry Tomatoes

Calories: 220 | Protein: 10g | Carbs: 15g | Fat: 14g

Dessert: Vanilla Bean Panna Cotta with Raspberry Coulis

Calories: 200 | Protein: 3g | Carbs: 30g | Fat: 8g

Beverage: Cold Brew Coffee with Vanilla Almond Milk

Calories: 30 | Protein: 1g | Carbs: 4g | Fat: 1g

Day 25:

Breakfast: Peanut Butter Banana Protein Pancakes

Calories: 320 | Protein: 15g | Carbs: 30g | Fat: 18g

Lunch: Quinoa and Roasted Vegetable Stuffed Peppers

Calories: 420 | Protein: 15g | Carbs: 60g | Fat: 18g

Dinner: Lemon Garlic Roasted Chicken with Rosemary Potatoes

Calories: 480 | Protein: 30g | Carbs: 35g | Fat: 22g

Snack: Hummus and Veggie Sticks

Calories: 150 | Protein: 5g | Carbs: 20g | Fat: 7g

Dessert: Pistachio and Raspberry Chocolate Bark

Calories: 150 | Protein: 3g | Carbs: 15g | Fat: 10g

Beverage: Pineapple Ginger Kombucha

Calories: 40 | Protein: 0g | Carbs: 10g | Fat: 0g

Day 26:

Breakfast: Berry-Licious Fruit Salad with Honey-Lime Drizzle

Calories: 90 | Protein: 1g | Carbs: 22g | Fat: 0g

Lunch: Caprese Stuffed Portobello Mushrooms

Calories: 350 | Protein: 12g | Carbs: 25g | Fat: 18g

Dinner: Butternut Squash and Sage Risotto

Calories: 410 | Protein: 10g | Carbs: 60g | Fat: 15g

Snack: Dark Chocolate-Dipped Strawberries

Calories: 120 | Protein: 1g | Carbs: 25g | Fat: 5g

Dessert: Coconut Chia Seed Pudding with Mango Puree

Calories: 180 | Protein: 4g | Carbs: 25g | Fat: 8g

Beverage: Sparkling Lavender Lemonade

Calories: 40 | Protein: 0g | Carbs: 10g | Fat: 0g

Day 27:

Breakfast: Blueberry Almond Overnight Oats

Calories: 280 | Protein: 10g | Carbs: 40g | Fat: 10g

Lunch: Tomato Basil Mozzarella Panini

Calories: 340 | Protein: 15g | Carbs: 35g | Fat: 16g

Dinner: Cauliflower Steak with Chimichurri Sauce

Calories: 370 | Protein: 15g | Carbs: 40g | Fat: 18g

Snack: Cheese and Whole Wheat Pita Wedges

Calories: 220 | Protein: 10g | Carbs: 15g | Fat: 14g

Dessert: Decadent Dark Chocolate Avocado Mousse

Calories: 150 | Protein: 3g | Carbs: 12g | Fat: 10g

Beverage: Pineapple Ginger Kombucha

Calories: 40 | Protein: 0g | Carbs: 10g | Fat: 0g

Day 28:

Breakfast: Spinach and Feta Omelette

Calories: 320 | Protein: 20g | Carbs: 15g | Fat: 22g

Lunch: Sweet Potato and Black Bean Quesadillas

Calories: 370 | Protein: 15g | Carbs: 40g | Fat: 18g

Dinner: Mushroom and Spinach Stuffed Chicken Breast

Calories: 380 | Protein: 35g | Carbs: 15g | Fat: 18g

Snack: Roasted Chickpeas with Paprika and Garlic

Calories: 160 | Protein: 6g | Carbs: 22g | Fat: 6g

Dessert: Classic Chocolate Chip Cookies

Calories: 120 | Protein: 2g | Carbs: 15g | Fat: 6g

Beverage: Sparkling Lavender Lemonade

Calories: 40 | Protein: 0g | Carbs: 10g | Fat: 0g

Day 29:

Breakfast: Chia Seed Pudding

Calories: 250 | Protein: 8g | Carbs: 30g | Fat: 12g

Lunch: Teriyaki Tofu Stir-Fry with Broccoli and Bell Peppers

Calories: 400 | Protein: 15g | Carbs: 35g | Fat: 18g

Dinner: Cilantro Lime Chicken Fajita Bowl

Calories: 380 | Protein: 25g | Carbs: 30g | Fat: 15g

Snack: Energy-boosting smoothie with Spinach and Banana

Calories: 230 | Protein: 12g | Carbs: 30g | Fat: 8g

Dessert: Pistachio and Raspberry Chocolate Bark

Calories: 150 | Protein: 3g | Carbs: 15g | Fat: 10g

Beverage: Raspberry Hibiscus Iced Tea

Calories: 20 | Protein: 0g | Carbs: 5g | Fat: 0g

Day 30:

Breakfast: Banana Nut Oatmeal

Calories: 290 | Protein: 10g | Carbs: 45g | Fat: 8g

Lunch: Mango Avocado Chicken Salad

Calories: 360 | Protein: 25g | Carbs: 30g | Fat: 16g

Dinner: Black Bean and Sweet Potato Enchiladas

Calories: 430 | Protein: 15g | Carbs: 50g | Fat: 20g

Snack: Whole Grain Crackers with Avocado and Cherry Tomatoes

Calories: 200 | Protein: 5g | Carbs: 20g | Fat: 12g

Dessert: Berry-Licious Fruit Salad with Honey-Lime Drizzle

Calories: 90 | Protein: 1g | Carbs: 22g | Fat: 0g

Beverage: Cold Brew Coffee with Vanilla Almond Milk

Calories: 30 | Protein: 1g | Carbs: 4g | Fat: 1g

Conclusion

Congratulations on concluding "The Congestive Heart Failure Diet Cookbook." This comprehensive guide has equipped you with valuable insights, practical tips, and delicious recipes to navigate the journey toward managing congestive heart failure through dietary choices.

Reflecting on a Heart-Healthy Journey

As we pause to reflect on the heart-healthy journey you've undertaken, it's essential to acknowledge the strides you've made and the transformative impact on your overall well-being. This reflection serves as a compass, guiding you through the milestones achieved, the challenges faced, and the continuous commitment to nurturing your heart health.

Celebrating Achievements:

Take a moment to celebrate the achievements, both big and small, on your heart-healthy journey. Whether it's consistently choosing nutrient-dense foods, incorporating regular exercise, or adopting mindful eating habits, each step contributes to your well-being.

Increased Awareness:

Reflect on the increased awareness you've gained regarding the nutritional choices that support heart health. From understanding the significance of key nutrients to making informed decisions while grocery shopping, your awareness has become a powerful tool in maintaining a heart-healthy lifestyle.

Culinary Exploration:

Consider the culinary exploration that has unfolded during this journey. Exploring new recipes, experimenting with flavors, and discovering the joy of preparing heart-healthy meals contribute not only to your physical health but also to a richer and more enjoyable relationship with food.

Lifestyle Integration:

Reflect on how heart-healthy practices have seamlessly integrated into your lifestyle. Whether it's the incorporation of daily physical activity, stress management techniques, or the mindful selection of ingredients, these practices are becoming a natural and integral part of your daily routine.

Navigating Challenges:

Acknowledge the challenges you've faced and how you've navigated through them. From moments of temptation to external pressures, your ability to stay committed to heart-healthy choices demonstrates resilience and a deep understanding of the importance of prioritizing your cardiovascular health.

Health and Vitality:

Take stock of improvements in your health and vitality. Whether it's increased energy levels, improved sleep, or a sense of overall well-being, these indicators are testimony to the positive impact of embracing a heart-healthy lifestyle.

Connection and Support:

Reflect on the connections forged and the support received during this journey. Whether from healthcare professionals, friends, or family, the strength of your support network plays a pivotal role in sustaining motivation and overcoming challenges.

Gratitude and Mindfulness:

Cultivate a sense of gratitude for the nourishment your body receives and the ability to make choices that support your heart health. Practicing mindfulness in your daily life further enhances the connection between your mind, body, and the nourishing choices you make.

Future Intentions:

As you reflect on the journey so far, set intentions for the future. Consider new goals, aspirations, and areas of focus that will continue to contribute to your heart-healthy lifestyle. The journey is ongoing, and each reflection informs the next step forward.

In this moment of reflection, honor the commitment you've shown to your heart health. Your journey is a testament to the power of conscious choices, resilience, and the transformative impact of prioritizing your cardiovascular well-being. May your reflections guide you toward continued growth, vitality, and a heart-healthy life.

Encouragement for Sustainable Change

Embarking on a journey of sustainable change is a commendable pursuit that requires determination, patience, and a steadfast commitment to your well-being. As you navigate this path towards a healthier and more heart-conscious lifestyle, consider these words of encouragement to fortify your spirit and reinforce your dedication to sustainable change.

Embrace Progress, Not Perfection:

Understand that sustainable change is a journey, not a destination. Embrace the progress you make, recognizing that small steps forward accumulate into significant transformations over time. Perfection is not the goal; progress is.

Celebrate Every Victory:

Take a moment to celebrate each victory, no matter how seemingly insignificant. Whether it's choosing a nutritious snack, completing a workout, or opting for a heart-healthy recipe, each positive choice contributes to the tapestry of your sustainable change.

Learn from Challenges:

Challenges are inevitable, but they are also invaluable teachers. View challenges as opportunities for growth and self-discovery. Learn from setbacks, adjust your course as needed, and use each challenge as a stepping stone toward resilience.

Cultivate Patience:

Sustainable change unfolds over time, requiring patience and persistence. Understand that lasting transformations don't happen overnight. Be patient with yourself, allowing the process to naturally evolve as you integrate heart-healthy practices into your lifestyle.

Build a Support System:

Surround yourself with a supportive network. Share your journey with friends, family, or a community that understands and encourages your goals. Having a strong support system motivates you during challenging moments and celebrates your achievements alongside you.

Focus on Nourishment, Not Deprivation:

Shift your mindset from deprivation to nourishment. Instead of dwelling on what you may be giving up, focus on the abundance of nourishing choices available. Embracing the positive aspects of your heart-healthy lifestyle makes sustainable change more fulfilling.

Prioritize Self-Care:

Sustainable change thrives in an environment of self-care. Prioritize your physical, emotional, and mental well-being. Ensure you get adequate rest, manage stress, and engage in activities that bring joy and relaxation. A well-nurtured self lays the foundation for lasting change.

Set Realistic Goals:

Set achievable and realistic goals. Break down larger objectives into smaller, manageable steps. This approach not only makes the journey less overwhelming but also allows you to celebrate victories along the way.
Adapt and Evolve:

Recognize that life is dynamic, and your journey may require adaptation. Be flexible and open to adjusting your approach as circumstances change. Sustainable change is about finding a rhythm that harmonizes with the ebb and flow of life.

Believe in Your Potential:

Lastly, believe in your potential for transformative change. You can shape your habits, prioritize your health, and create a sustainable and heart-healthy lifestyle. Trust in your ability to make choices that nurture not only your heart but your overall well-being.
As you embark on this journey of sustainable change, remember that every positive choice is a step toward a healthier, more fulfilling life. Be kind to

yourself, stay focused on your goals, and take pride in the sustainable changes you're making for a heart-healthy future.

A Final Note

As we arrive at the closing pages of this culinary and health companion, consider this final note not as an endpoint but as a meaningful pause in the ongoing narrative of your well-being. Your journey through the "Congestive Heart Failure Diet Cookbook" has been a tapestry of exploration, discovery, and conscious choices. Here, in this concluding moment, let's reflect on the essence of your experience and the possibilities that lie ahead.

Express gratitude for the journey you've undertaken. Gratitude not only for the nourishment your body has received but for the commitment you've shown to understanding and embracing a heart-healthy lifestyle.

Your journey has been a symphony of flavors, a culinary exploration that transcends the mere act of eating. It's an embrace of nourishment, a celebration of the senses, and a realization that wholesome, heart-healthy meals can be both flavorful and fulfilling.

Armed with knowledge about the mechanisms of congestive heart failure, dietary guidelines, and an array of heart-healthy recipes, you stand empowered. Knowledge is the compass that guides sustainable change, and you now hold that compass firmly in your hands.

Sustainable change is not a destination; it's a lifestyle. As you reflect on the recipes tried, the nutritional principles learned, and the lifestyle adjustments made, recognize that each choice is a step toward a healthier and more vibrant life.

The concluding pages of this cookbook mark a crossroads where reflection meets anticipation. Your heart-healthy journey continues beyond these words. Embrace the opportunities to explore new recipes, refine your culinary skills, and continually evolve your understanding of what it means to live heart-consciously.

Acknowledge the importance of support and community. Whether you've shared this journey with loved ones or found encouragement within a community, know that you are not alone. The strength of shared experiences propels us forward.

Your commitment to heart-healthy lifestyle matters—not only for your cardiovascular health but as an inspiration to those around you. Your choices ripple beyond your well-being, creating a positive impact on the broader tapestry of health and wellness.

Life, like a well-crafted dish, is a blend of diverse flavors. Embrace the sweetness of achievements, the richness of experiences, and the depth of lessons learned. Your heart-healthy journey is not just about physical health; it's about savoring the richness of life itself.

As we conclude this chapter, remember that your story is ongoing. The pages turn, and with each chapter, you have the opportunity to shape a narrative of vibrant health, mindful choices, and a heart that beats with resilience and vitality. May your future be filled with the continued exploration of flavors, the joy of nourishing choices, and the fulfillment that comes from living a heart-healthy life. With warm wishes on your continued journey, The Congestive Heart Failure Diet Cookbook Team